Tea Cleanse

The Ultimate Beginner's Guide & Action Plan to Tea Cleansing Diet for Weight Loss – A Natural Solution to Detox & Boost Your Body's Metabolism

By Jennifer Louissa

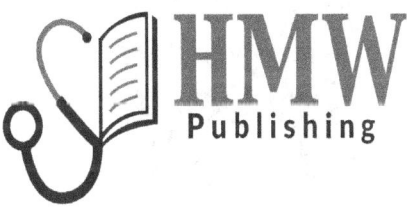

For more great books visit:

HMWPublishing.com

Get another book for free

I want to thank you for purchasing this book and offer you another book (just as long and valuable as this book), "Health & Fitness Mistakes You Don't Know You're Making", completely free.

Visit the link below to signup and receive it:

www.hmwpublishing.com/gift

In this book, I will break down the most common health & fitness mistakes, you are probably committing right now, and I will reveal how you can easily get in the best shape of your life!

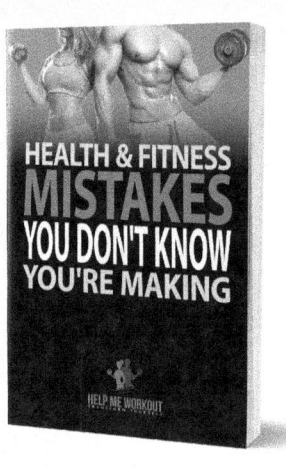

In addition to this valuable gift, you will also have an opportunity to get our new books for free, enter giveaways, and receive other valuable emails from me. Again, visit the link to sign up:

www.hmwpublishing.com/gift

Table Of Content

Book Description 7

Introduction 9

Chapter 1: What are Toxins? 12

    The Different Sources of Toxins 14

    How do Toxins Affect You? 18

Chapter 2: Tea Cleansing in a Nutshell 19

    True Tea for Cleansing? 20

    Builds Your Immune System 23

    Curbs Your Appetite 23

    Helps the Body in Digestion 25

    What Happens Inside Your Body During Cleansing 25

    Important Suggestions Before Starting Tea Cleansing 26

Chapter 3: The Truth About Tea Bags

....29

Chapter 4: Best Type of Teas for Cleansing

....35

Chapter 5: The Benefits of Tea Cleansing

....39

- Green Tea: 40
- Black Tea: 40
- Darjeeling Tea: 41
- Blooming Tea: 41
- White Tea: 42

Chapter 6: Proper Tea Brewing 44

- Water 44
- Type of Teapots......................................45
- Steep Times and Temperature 46
- Guidelines 47

Chapter 7: Grading Your Tea Leaves .52

Chapter 8: How Do You Choose the Proper Tea for Detoxing 58

Full or Broken Leaf Tea? 58

What are the Tea Benefits You are After? 59

Chapter 9: Cleansing Plan 67

Chapter 10: Reminders and Take-Aways 71

Conclusion 77

Final Words 79

Book Description

There have been a lot of trips to the gym and never have they ended up in your daily life routine. The gym is good until your school starts again or your boss starts giving you more work, and you realize there is no time for it in your tight routine, and you feel the unnecessary fat under your touch.

The diet plans are stuck in your fridge and trying them has been hard. Eating vegetables and fruits are fun until you feel the lethargy and weakness kick in. It isn't too late when you feel the mood swings coming right at you, and a little too soon, you find yourself eating the greasy food from the nearest junk food place. Reading this, you will know an easy way to lose weight and flush out the toxins.

There is nothing saddening than feeling helpless and not being able to do anything about it. This book will take you step by step and enlighten you about an amazing way to lose weight, and you will be more than happy to use it.

In this book, you will be told about:

- What are toxins and how they are harmful to your body

- What problems you face while losing weight.

- If the toxins stay in your body, how they harm you.

- Cleansing tea is a very simple way to lose weight and fasten your metabolism.

INTRODUCTION

If there is one thing that we do not know about toxins, it is that having them inside our bodies in a certain amount can make it enough for them to earn the label *harmful*.

True enough there are so many ways that different toxins affect us, but one of the most known effects they have is us getting fat. Many of these toxins enter our system as an ingredient of some unhealthy food that we blatantly choose.

Undoubtedly, most of us already went through the phase where we only choose to blame other people and things. Admit it, many of us think that blaming anything other than yourself makes it more comfortable, but think again. Regardless of who you are accusing, it will still not make your health any better.

So, we move on to your sudden urge to finally put things right and tea cleansing, together with other healthy options, suddenly enter the scene. But what is tea cleansing? Is it a viable option to keep trim or does it only cleanse you from the inside? Let us delve deeper into the facts about tea cleansing; you will soon find out why the old world appreciated it so much. Thanks again for purchasing this book, I hope you reading enjoy it and please do not forget to leave us an honest review 😊!

Also, before you get started, I recommend you joining our email newsletter to receive updates on any upcoming new book releases or promotions. You can sign-up for free, and as a bonus, you will receive a free gift. Our "*Health & Fitness Mistakes You Don't Know You're Making*" book! This book has been written to demystify, expose the top do's and don'ts and to finally equip you with the information you need to get in the best shape of your life. Due to the overwhelming amount of mis-information and lies told by magazines and self-proclaimed "gurus", it's becoming harder and harder to get reliable information to get in shape. As opposed to having to go through dozens of biased, unreliable and un-trustworthy sources to get

INTRODUCTION

If there is one thing that we do not know about toxins, it is that having them inside our bodies in a certain amount can make it enough for them to earn the label *harmful*.

True enough there are so many ways that different toxins affect us, but one of the most known effects they have is us getting fat. Many of these toxins enter our system as an ingredient of some unhealthy food that we blatantly choose.

Undoubtedly, most of us already went through the phase where we only choose to blame other people and things. Admit it, many of us think that blaming anything other than yourself makes it more comfortable, but think again. Regardless of who you are accusing, it will still not make your health any better.

So, we move on to your sudden urge to finally put things right and tea cleansing, together with other healthy options, suddenly enter the scene. But what is tea cleansing? Is it a viable option to keep trim or does it only cleanse you from the inside? Let us delve deeper into the facts about tea cleansing; you will soon find out why the old world appreciated it so much. Thanks again for purchasing this book, I hope you reading enjoy it and please do not forget to leave us an honest review 😊 !

Also, before you get started, I recommend you [joining our email newsletter](#) to receive updates on any upcoming new book releases or promotions. You can sign-up for free, and as a bonus, you will receive a free gift. Our "*Health & Fitness Mistakes You Don't Know You're Making*" book! This book has been written to demystify, expose the top do's and don'ts and to finally equip you with the information you need to get in the best shape of your life. Due to the overwhelming amount of mis-information and lies told by magazines and self-proclaimed "gurus", it's becoming harder and harder to get reliable information to get in shape. As opposed to having to go through dozens of biased, unreliable and un-trustworthy sources to get your health & fitness information. Everything you need to help you has been broken down in this book for you to easily follow and to immediately get results to achieve your desired fitness goals in the shortest amount of time.

Once again, to join our free email newsletter and to receive a free copy of this valuable book, please visit the link and signup now: **www.hmwpublishing.com/gift**

CHAPTER 1: WHAT ARE TOXINS?

We have been hearing the word *toxins* for such a long time that we have learned to either ignore its true meaning or not even try to find out what it means.

For many, toxins are the things that our body naturally excrete as a part of cleansing and protecting itself. That can be quite right, but that does not precisely answer the what part.

Toxins are harmful agents that can be environmental, biological, and even autogenous. Meaning they from the environment (air, water, the food we eat, and also the chemicals we use in our daily lives) or from the byproducts of our bodies. These things do not cause anything else but harm. In short, they are poison to us. As for autogenous toxins, these are the toxins that we are born with that stems from the generations of toxins that our family is exposed to.

It is also good for you to know that toxins do not only poison your body, they also poison your mind. How so? They creep into your system gently; you will not even feel it until it is already too late. First, they affect your body slowly, hindering it from functioning well. This effect alone can already lead to stress, what with our body trying to find a way to operate as it should, add to that your frustration that lately, you keep on feeling that something is off.

Stress does not only impede you from doing your daily work and from your body to function regularly, but it also ruins your usual pattern, and if left unattended, can lead to burn out. Burn out will not kill you. What will kill you are the complications that it exposes you to. You see, when a person is burned out, his or her immune system goes down and exposes you to a high risk of contracting diseases. That disease you are exposed to will eventually kill you. I'm quite sure nobody wants that to happen to them.

These poisons also have different forms and sources, roughly reaching up to 600 variations, give or take a few. With a list of poisons such as this you can, pretty much, say that almost everything around you contains toxins. So, what does eating have to do with them?

Watching our food intake helps us reduce the toxins that enter or get produced in our bodies. Let me be clear though, watching what we eat does not help us too much with expelling the poisons from our system. The only way for us to discharge these harmful things is by urinating and defecating. As for the belief that sweat helps out in removing them, not really. You can run all day or find a way to sweat excessively. Yes, you will slim down, but the toxins will still be there.

THE DIFFERENT SOURCES OF TOXINS

Air - Toxins from air enter through our skin and lungs.

- Any burning organic compound* is already a toxin because it produces tar that travels through the airway and eventually damages the lungs. A good example is a tar from smoking or second-hand smoking, joystick smoke as a relaxant for massages, yoga sessions, and even tai chi classes.

- Ammonia that can be found in animal urine that has been standing for days or cigarettes.

- Chemical cleaning products especially those with

strong fumes like bleach or muriatic acid.

- Chemical spray such as air fresheners.

- Fumes from fireworks, petrochemical-based products, nail lacquers, hair spray, airplane cabin air, traffic fumes, printer inks, and more.

*organic compound – any solid, liquid, or gaseous compound that contains carbon in its molecules.

Water (not ingested) - Toxins from water enter through our eyes, skin, and air.

- Chlorine, chloroform, hydrogen sulfide, and trichloroethylene that can be absorbed while bathing, especially with hot showers that strip off our body's natural oils and exposes our pores.

- Chloramines, trichloramine, trihalomethanes, and other ammonium compounds (urine, lotion, oil from the skin, flakes from dry skin) that can be absorbed when bathing in ponds, lakes, rivers, and the sea.

Water (ingested)

- Fluoride, chlorine, cadmium from tap water, mineral water, and well water.

- Food

- Including beverages made from powdered juice, coffee, tea, or fruits and vegetables sprayed with chemicals by the growers.

- Additives, food colouring, monosodium glutamate (MSG), preservatives, artificial flavouring, artificial sweeteners and more that can be found on your regular store-bought food.

Chemicals

- Medicines such as antibiotics.

- Vaccines containing mercury or thimerosal (organic mercury).

- Tattoo ink contains mercury.

- Amalgam fillings containing mercury.

- Shampoo, conditioner, makeup, lotion, mouthwash containing preservatives like paraben, propylparaben, ethylparaben, methylparaben that can trigger your cancer cells. Sulfates, the preservation and foaming agents that cause allergy-like symptoms such as difficulty in breathing or hives. PEG or polyethylene glycol, a thickener, softener, or moisture carrier that reduces the natural moisture of your skin leaving you more exposed to bacteria.

PEG or polyethylene glycol, when indicated on the label for ingredients, is usually followed by a bunch of numbers like PEG-40 or PEG-150. The higher the number that follows the acronym PEG, the safer it is, because the lower number means it is a lot easier for your skin to absorb it.

Good to know: *The human body is exposed to about 200 types of organic chemicals daily due to the intake of food and its additives, the use of cleaning products, toiletries, and even makeup.*

How do Toxins Affect You?

The truth is that there are many products and things we use in our everyday lives that contain chemicals. These chemicals are all potentially toxic, and once they reach a certain level, that is when they can affect you. How so? Depends on the dosage or the amounts of it that we have in our body. Add to that the fact that we either choose to ignore or do not take caution to their ultimate effects because, well, we do not see them.

We, humans, are used to recognizing harm only when we can see it large and looming right in front of our eyes. Until then, everything seems to go swimmingly for us even if the truth says otherwise.

Chapter 2: Tea Cleansing in a Nutshell

Tea cleansing, for many, is a method of drinking "*dieting or slimming*" tea, fasting, and avoiding a whole bunch of food groups to get the "*toxins*" out of their system that will hasten their slimming down.

This is not how your tea cleansing will go. In fact, nobody's tea cleansing method should go like that, because it is dangerous for your health. You will be using true teas and **tisanes** or herbal teas instead. You will not be forcing your body to do anything. All that you will be doing is gently introducing healthy things into your body, and encouraging it to cleanse your system for it to function well.

Just to be clear, we are not talking about this dieting or slimming tea. We are talking about the true teas and the herbal ones that indeed give you health benefits.

TRUE TEA FOR CLEANSING?

So, herbal teas are known to be used for tea cleansing; there is no problem with that. But true teas? Is there such thing – cleansing with true teas?

Yes, there is such thing. Trust me. Before I even started with loose leaves (by the way, let me tell you that if you start going for loose leaves, you will not go back), I used to consume true tea in teabags, just because I wanted to. I did not intend to get slimmer; I just want to feel warmer and lessen my coffee consumption. I had this fixation with Earl Grey; it is a kind of black tea.

Two weeks passed, I still drink my Earl Grey a cup or two daily. Then I noticed my metabolism became better, like everyday-bowel-movement kind of better. Some of my clothes that chafed did not chafe anymore. All my clothes are a comfortable fit. I slept better, plus I felt lighter, never bloated. And that was just a two-week consumption of black tea. Imagine doing that using green tea.

Plus, come on, if true tea is not for tea cleansing, then how do you explain the ridiculously long lives of the old Chinese people and other East Asians who did nothing but drink tea? They drink tea in the morning, at noon, in the evening, during and after meals, drink it just for fun, when sick, in birthdays and all the time. Tea is like water for them, and that is saying something because they consume true tea.

First things first, you have to know that we have options for the kind of tea that you want to use. Our tea options are green tea, black tea, white tea, oolong, rooibos, peppermint, Darjeeling, dandelion tea, and other blooming teas.

With all these options, your body goes on a natural detoxification, without you having to force it to go to that mode. It would be a good thing for you to know that forcing your body to go to detox mode is quite dangerous, so doing that is out of the question.

Your detoxification will take place naturally. It will not impede you from your daily activities; you do not need to fast or go hungry altogether. All you need to do is drink your tea daily, watch your food portioning, throw in a bit of exercise, and all is well. In fact, you can even drink the tea just because you want to drink it. Just enjoy it and while your body is gradually healing and protecting itself.

You do not need to wait for a whole day off from work so that you can drink your tea and worry about a rumbling stomach and annoying toilet sessions for the rest of the day. That is not going to happen with these classic tea options.

BUILDS YOUR IMMUNE SYSTEM

You will find that regardless of the type or flavour of the tea you use for cleansing, they are all good for your immune system because they can strengthen it.

All of the classic herbal teas contain an antioxidant that is highly beneficial to your body, especially the black, white, and green tea.

CURBS YOUR APPETITE

Yes, teas can curb your appetite. While there is some tea that specializes in this function naturally, it would be good for you to know that teas, in general, are useful in curbing your appetite. It makes you feel fuller longer than before you drank your tea. You know why?

Catechins! With lots of antioxidants that you can find in all of these natural teas, surely catechin is one of the antioxidants it contains. It encourages your body to use up your extra fat storage, so, it is all good for you.

However, another good thing that catechins do is balancing your blood sugar. It does so by slowing down the elevation of your blood sugar levels. How?

You see, sugar to travel in our system, needs to be bound to a blood cell. Once it goes in our system and gets to a certain high level, the insulin in our pancreas gets triggered. Insulin will then, start using those sugar in our blood and converts them into energy for us to use or, if we have enough energy, stores them so that insulin can easily turn them for future use once our energy runs out.

That whole process is being slowed down by catechins, in turn, you get blood (without sugar) that circulates in your system while sugar is being held under control by catechins. With tea drinking, your threshold for energy to be used becomes increased, encouraging your body to use its fat reserves. Then it slows down the binding of sugar to your blood, efficiently keeping your blood sugar and insulin levels in balance. If your blood sugar is balanced, your body will not ask your brain to signal you for food supply.

HELPS THE BODY IN DIGESTION

Teas help your body because they have these anti-inflammatory properties that protect your digestive system from being upset. Drinking it hot also aids in cleaning your gut.

If you put an oily food inside the fridge and you see the oil start to solidify, that is pretty much what happens inside your gut if you love eating greasy foods and then drinking something cold afterward. So, regular drinking of hot tea gradually cleanses your stomach of this muck, resulting in smoother digestion. Plus, if you drink hot tea after a meal, it helps with the absorption a lot faster.

WHAT HAPPENS INSIDE YOUR BODY DURING CLEANSING

Well, apart from better digestion or curbing your hunger, drinking tea encourages sweating. And no, you are not sweating because your body is getting rid of the toxins in it.

You are sweating because your body is trying to cool down, to keep everything inside your body working flawlessly. If you drink something cold, your body will try to cope by making more heat; however, if you drink something hot or warm, your body will deal with it by **regulating** the temperature inside it that often results to you feeling colder. Such bonus.

And so, drinking hot tea in summer is not such a bad idea. This explains why tea drinkers often feel refreshed after a cup of hot tea, as opposed to drinking something cold that makes them more thirsty.

Tea also burns calories with the help of caffeine. Caffeine encourages your body to use more energy resulting in more calories being consumed in the process.

Important Suggestions Before Starting Tea Cleansing

As opposed to the popular method people use when tea

cleansing such as fasting, our tea cleansing method focuses on the natural methods. It just makes sense because we will be using what we call true teas or that tea that come from the plant *Camellia Sinensis* and other herbs that produce, not dieting or slimming teas that are already processed and added with unknown and weird ingredients.

1. Eat, never starve yourself.

You do not need to avoid a whole food group. All you need is *avoid processed food* as much as possible. This includes junk food, anything with MSG or monosodium glutamate, soda, processed meat.

In cases where you cannot avoid them, make sure you keep to your tea drinking routine to help your body get rid of the toxins it got from such foods.

Also, never even try to fast. You do not need to fast for the tea to start helping your body with the detoxification and other processes. Plus, going hungry will just ruin your metabolism yet, again.

2. Do not drink your tea cold.

Unless you just want to drink it without being concerned about the benefits that hot tea can give you. You see, tea that is left too long until it has gone cold does not taste as good anymore. Plus, hot water just brings out the best in tea such as your antioxidants.

3. Choose your tea well.

Choose which tea is best for you. It can be the flavour or the benefits. The one that you love most works best.

Chapter 3: The Truth About Tea Bags

Ah, one thing that tea purists will insist is that loose leaf teas are better. Then again, tea bags are cheaper, plus it gives you the same good stuff, and flavour, right?

Not exactly. I hate to burst that practicality bubble of yours but there is more to tea bags than just tea, and often, it does not mean good news.

Whenever watching a Japanese or Chinese movie, or any movie that involves the East Asian culture, at one point, you will see them pouring a pot of tea for a guest. So, let me ask you something. Have you ever seen them dipping a tea bag in the teapot for steeping? No, right?

That is because initially, tea is being enjoyed by boiling the leaves - like full, actual plant leaves. Those leaves swell a little, then get soggy and wilted when being boiled. This straightforward and seemingly dull process means a lot when it comes to tea.

Now, imagine suppressing that little leaf-swelling phase of the tea leaves inside a tea bag while boiling them. Ha! It does nothing! – Not really.

You see, tea manufacturers place their premium teas in a can. Inside that can are loose leaves, NOT INDIVIDUALLY-WRAPPED BAGS. And they call it the premium for a reason. Those tea leaves in the can are whole leaves, not broken, not powdered or crushed. These cans mostly go to different tea stores, not in the supermarket.

Now, when you have picked all the whole tea leaves from the bunch, placed them in their beautiful cans, you are left with broken leaves and crushed powdered leaves. Some of those broken leaves go inside beautiful cans as well but are being sold cheaper than the full-leafed ones. Most of these cans go to the supermarket to be sold.

So, with the full leaves tea in their cans, the broken leaves in their cans as well, you are left with crushed minuscule leaves, dust, and powdered tea. They go inside little tea bags that are, then, individually wrapped, placed in boxes, and straight they go to the supermarket. They are the cheapest of the bunch.

Another method for manufacturers to produce mass tea (high volume, low quality) is through the use of a machine that uses the CTC method, or Crush-Torn-Curl, to produce pellets formed out of tea leaves. These pellets are then placed inside the teabags, et voila! You now have your cheap tea.

So, what's the problem with their packaging?

Well, tea leaves have tannins. Tannins give tea the astringent properties and the bitter flavour. Some contain low amounts of it like white tea and green tea.

Now, when full leaf teas are boiled, tannins get released a couple of seconds after. This gives the tea that slight aroma kick and a little bitterness, but that's all good. If your full leaf tea does not give you this little bit of bitterness or astringent feel when boiling it, it might mean it is low quality or old stock. The same story goes for broken tea leaves, except, the tannins create a bit more bitter taste to the tea.

As for the powdered left-over tea leaves, if you accidentally forgot that you are steeping it, left it in there a tad bit longer, once you drink it do not be surprised if you get that medicine-like bitterness from your supposedly lovely cup of tea. Because that is the consequences of crushed tea, it has more tannins than you would want and even if you steep it carefully, you will still get a bitter taste.

Add to that the fact that even if there is a whole bit of tea leaf that got accidentally included in the tea bag, the leaves are still there stuck in that packet. The tea bag will never let them float and get the water they need to expand and bring out the true smell and flavour of the tea.

Then again, if you are not the type who cares so much about the taste of your tea, or you just love its bitter taste, then you would think that it should be no problem at all, right?

Again, not really. This is because apart from more tannins being released from tea bags and less flavour, you also get fewer benefits.

Those antioxidants and catechins I mentioned in the previous chapters? You are likely not going to get them from these tea bags. This is because once a tea leaf has been crushed or broken, the essential oils that it contains that helps create the flavour and scent, are lost. Whatever is left in that tea bag of yours are remnants of the tea leaf's full-flavoured glory.

So, what to do now? What if you still want to save up and you do not want to stock on big canisters of loose leaf teas, or you just want to try a flavour and such?

Well, I suggest that you go for those companies that produce pyramid-shaped tea bags. They are a tad bit expensive than your regular bland-tasting tea bags, but it's going to give you a good taste test for the full-leafed ones in the can.

Pyramid-shaped tea bags have a bigger room that allows the leaves to swim when dipped in boiling water. This enables the leaves to expand and release the flavour. What's more, they also contain full leaves or broken leaves at worst. But that's it, no crushed or powdered leaves.

Chapter 4: Best Type of Teas for Cleansing

1. **Green, Black, and White Tea**

For the green, black, and white tea, what you have to remember about them is the ingredient call catechin.

Catechins are antioxidants. First, antioxidants. We take Vitamin C for this reason, we need antioxidants, and we have no other choice but to find an external source for this particular component because the body cannot produce it on its own. Antioxidants help strengthen your immunity system, protects you from common illnesses and frightening diseases as well such as cardiovascular diseases and cancer.

That being said, of course, we all want the antioxidant and one type of it is what we call catechins found in black, white, and green tea. So you drink tea like it is a regular, uncomplicated day, and you now have your antioxidant. Easy just like that. The good thing about catechins is that it does not only keep you safe from a myriad of illnesses and continues to protect you, they are also the one responsible for creating the flavour in your tea and other drinks like wine.

Now, let us focus on the catechins found in tea. What does it do? It helps you slim down by *increasing the allowed amount* of energy that your body can use than its usual amount. This way, all those sitting fats in our bodies, waiting for forever to be used, are *finally* converted into energy and then put to use. This results in weight loss.

2. Oolong Tea

Oolong tea, on the other hand, has so many antioxidants and it mostly works by boosting your metabolism. So, if you have a problem with your daily morning business, might as well choose oolong tea to regulate that before you move on to slimming down.

3. Rooibos Tea

For rooibos tea, well, if you are entirely new to tea drinking or you are a sweet tooth, you will appreciate this tea better than the other ones. You see, rooibos is a tad sweet without you having to add anything to it. You get to enjoy the natural sweetness without worries, plus you also get the benefits of its component, **aspalathin**. Aspalathin helps you curb your stress-induced hunger by reducing your stress hormones. So, no more stress eating.

4. Peppermint Tea

Peppermint tea is obviously peppermint flavoured, so if you are a lover of anything that has to do with this specific flavour, you are always free to choose this tea. The good thing about this is that it suppresses your appetite, no additional ingredients to be added. It is just that, all natural. Also, it is a little sweet, so it is indeed a treat to those who are cutting back on sugar to keep healthy.

5. Dandelion Tea

Dandelion tea is a natural diuretic. Meaning it will encourage your liver to keep processing the water in your body and eliminate it, including toxins. If you suffer from heartburn, then this is an excellent natural treatment for you to keep it at bay. It also helps you balance your blood glucose levels.

Chapter 5: The Benefits of Tea Cleansing

Detoxing has been one of the many fads lately, inspired by celebrities who have so much money, they do not even know which thing they are spending their money on is keeping them trim. They just show you they are trim.

Then again, many studies and research have already exposed the not-so-good side of detoxing. This is where tea cleansing comes in. It is a lot easier approach to keeping healthy and trim than the bothersome detoxing.

So, apart from the fact that tea lowers your risk of stroke, heart disease, reduce your blood pressure, increase your mood and mental performance, what else does it do?

Well, like mentioned earlier, it boosts your energy. In effect, it helps prevent you from gaining extra and unwanted weight.

Green Tea:

Usually in packed leaves or powder form. Matcha, a type of green tea, contains five times more L-theanine than the usual green tea.

L-theanine is a component that can be found in teas taken from Camellia Sinensis. It helps give relaxation without making you feel drowsy.

- Antibacterial
- Fights diabetes
- Prevents dementia
- Lowers cholesterol levels
- Fights bad breath
- Helps reduce stress
- Strengthens teeth

Black Tea:

The type of tea that contains high levels of anti-oxidants.

(Assam, Earl Grey, Darjeeling, Keemun, Yunan, Ceylon, Bai lin)

- Highly effective in flushing out the toxins in your body
- Has more antioxidants than any other teas, which is vital in preventing cancer

DARJEELING TEA:

Another type of black tea

- Helps calm and soothe your mind
- Has high antioxidant

BLOOMING TEA:

The flashiest of all the teas. Very beautiful to look at, blooms while steeping in water. (Dandelion, Coriander, Cardamom, Cinnamon, Jasmine, Licorice, Ginger, and Sage)

- Helps your metabolism, makes it function smoothly
- Lowers cholesterol
- Balances blood sugar levels
- Gets rid of halitosis or bad breath
- Strengthens and cleans the digestive tract
- Improves immune system
- Helps reduce GERD or acid reflux
- Calms the irritation in your stomach's lining
- Diuretic (

WHITE TEA:

Made from the youngest Camellia Sinensis leaves.

- Contains more antioxidants as compared to Green Tea
- Has anti-aging properties to slow down the process of wrinkling skin

- Protects you from UV rays

- Helps people with diabetes from excessive thirst and increased secretion of insulin

- Helps maintain your reproductive health in good condition

Chapter 6: Proper Tea Brewing

Let us say that you have already chosen your tea, what's next? You are going to make your tea now. Surely you know how to boil water, and you think it is just that easy. Well, it could be, if you do not care about how your tea is going to taste and if your brewing style will bring out the best components in it – that is unless you are a professional tea sommelier.

Water

Best option: Spring or Purified water.

The best water to use for steeping tea is purified or spring water because they do not contain pollutants that can change the taste of the tea. If your water is rich in natural minerals, chances are it will bring out better flavours of your tea.

You may think opting for distilled water is good, but dead water brings out bland or flat tasting tea, nobody likes that.

As for boiled tap water, it is also not a good option for tea brewing. Because it might have already been contaminated by the substances that are flowing in the water pipes and it can positively alter the tea's taste.

Type of Teapots

You know how water can affect the taste of tea? The same can be said for the teapot that you use. So, you do not just go to a tea shop and grab some random teapot to deal with it. If you genuinely want to bring out the best flavours and benefits of your tea, you will have to brew it right. Meaning the water, the duration of brewing, water temperature, and the pot should be the right ones because those things I just mentioned contribute to the result of the tea.

So, for you to have the teapot, you must first have your tea or at least know which tea you are buying the teapot for.

Teas that need high temperatures to bring out the best flavours are best partnered with teapots that are good in retaining heat. On the other hand, teas that need to be brewed at lower temperatures need teapots that will release heat in order not to over brewing them.

Now, there are light teapots, and there are ones that are quite heavy. The ones that are heavy are usually the ones that are good at retaining heat. So you buy them if you choose to have black tea or pu-erh (fermented) tea. On the other hand, tea that is more delicate and can easily get ruined through over brewing, like white or green tea, needs a teapot that can release the heat. This means glass or porcelain teapots is your best option for such tea.

STEEP TIMES AND TEMPERATURE

If there is anything that you need to put in mind when it comes to brewing tea, that would be this:

Each type of tea has a specific temperature level required for you to brew it properly.

The one-size fits all principle do not apply to the water for tea brewing. Following the correct water temperature for each type of tea will help you bring out its best flavour and benefits.

With temperature level, also comes the length of time the tea should be steeped. Again, the one-size fits all principle does not apply here. Before this chapter ends, I will give you a list of the steep times and proper temperature. Then again, once you have tried to follow the correct steep time for your chosen tea and you feel like it is too weak or strong for you, you can always follow your heart to get the right amount of flavour you want. As it is, we will first start walking before we run, or you risk wasting those precious tea leaves.

Guidelines

1. Make sure you have your purified water or freshly drawn spring water. Prepare the teapots and the teacups as well.

2. Let the water boil gently in a kettle.

(Gentle boil means when you look at the water when you think it is already boiling, there is a gentle, yet steady stream of bubbles on the surface. We are not after the angry kind of boiling water where the bubbles start to occupy the whole kettle and starts to look like it is going to come out and chase you anytime soon.)

3. Now, gently pour the hot water into the teapot. Pour some boiling water into each teacup as well. This is to warm the cups so that when you and your friends or family start drinking the tea, you get to enjoy the consistency of flavour because of the cup temperature.

4. Add the tea leaves, making sure you measure it <u>based on the number of people that will drink the tea</u>.

5. Let the water cool until it reaches the suggested temperature for the tea and then adds the tea leaves.

6. Let the water cool until it reaches the suggested temperature for the tea and then add the tea

leaves.

7. Now, remember your steeping time. It depends on which tea leaves you are using. Steep the tea based on the correct steeping time, wait, and time it. You should be as precise as you can.

8. Once the tea has steeped correctly, you can strain or transfer it to another serving teapot or pour it directly into the teacups.

Tea	Measurcment	Steep Time	Temperature	Teapot
Black Tea Full Leaf	1-2 teaspoons	2-3 minutes	203°F	Porcelain
Broken Leaf	1-2 teaspoons	3-5 minutes	203°F	Porcelain

Green Tea Chinese	2 teaspoons	2-3 minutes	176° - 185°F	Glass/ Porcelain
Japanese	1-2 teaspoons	3-5 minutes	203°F	Glass/ Earthenware
Oolong Tea Light (Green)	2-3 teaspoons	2-3 minutes	185° - 203°F	Porcelain/ Yixing Porcelain
Heavy (Dark)	3-2 teaspoons	3-5 minutes	203°F	
Pu-Erh Tea	1-2 teaspoons	3 minutes	212°F	Yixing
Tisanes (Herbal Tea)	1-2 teaspoons	3 minutes	212°F	Glass/ Porcelain

White Tea	2-3 teaspoons	3 minutes	176° - 185°F	Glass/ Porcelain

Chapter 7: Grading Your Tea Leaves

How tea leaves graded? We base it on the traditional preparation or processing of tea leaves in China. After all, that is where it all started.

Then again, it would be good for you to know that the Chinese people themselves understand the proper processing of tea leaves by heart, but do not label the process as such. Grading of tea leaves is used in countries such as Sri Lanka or India, anywhere in the world except China.

Now, why is grading important? If you value your health so much and you intend to give your body the best tea that your money can buy, you will have to have an inkling about tea grading. Either that or you just make your way to the store, buy your whole tea leaves, and you're done. That method does not work for everyone, though.

To those who prefer precision and knowing their money's worth. Here are the categories for grading the leaves:

1. Size – Are the tea leaves big or small? Are they full or broken?

    For this category, small, full leaves are preferred because it means younger leaves are used.

2. What kind of tea leaves are used? Is it made of young leaves or mature ones?

    The younger the leaves, the more delicate tea it yields. If you see tips or small whole leaves, that means you might just have the best bunch of leaves from the entire plant. Seeing the tips from a bunch of processed tea indicates sweet notes once it is brewed. The tips have all the nutrients as well.

Full Leaf Teas

OP (Orange Pekoe)	Consists of the top two leaves
FOP (Flowery Orange Pekoe)	Made from the tips and top two leaves
GFOP (Golden Flowery Orange Pekoe)	Has more tips proportion than FOP
TGFOP (Tippy Golden Flowery Orange Pekoe)	Has more tips proportion than GFOP
FTGFOP (Finest Tippy Golden Flowery Orange Pekoe)	High-quality FOP
STGFOP (Special Finest Tippy Golden Flower Orange Pekoe)	Best quality FOP

*If the grade is added with '1' at the end (FOP1 or STGFOP1), it means that it is the finest quality within that grade.

Broken:	Means the leaves are broken and will be used for bagged teas.
Orange:	Not about tea flavour. Orange may suggest the association of tea to the House of Orange when it became popular in the west. May also pertains to the colour of the leaf. A high-quality tea leaf turns into a copper colour when fully oxidized.
Pekoe or Orange Pekoe:	Uncertain origin. Used to describe the presence of tips or budding leaf found on the tea plant.

Tips:	Unopened leaves of the plant.
Tippy:	Teas with the presence of tips from younger leaves are labeled with the term "tippy."

Broken Leaf Teas

BOP (Broken Orange Pekoe)	Consists of broken top two leaves
FBOP (Flowery Broken Orange Pekoe)	Made from the tips and top two broken leaves
GBOP (Golden Broken Orange Pekoe)	Has more tips proportion than FOP, broken
TGBOP (Tippy Golden Broken Orange Pekoe)	Has more tips proportion than GBOP, broken

| GFBOP (Golden Flowery Broken Orange Pekoe) | Best quality FBOP |

Chapter 8: How Do You Choose the Proper Tea for Detoxing

Now that you know the grading, it is time for you to choose the proper tea for you. So, do you prefer full leaf tea or broken tea?

Full or Broken Leaf Tea?

Choosing full leaf tea will mean you have the more delicate tea, they are expensive and promises the true flavour of that type of tea that you want. However, that would also mean you will have to steep them longer because full leaves take longer to steep. They promise the true flavour of the tea, but it will be subtle. Subtle flavours are good if you love how they hint you with the different notes of the tea leaves. It keeps you wanting for more without overwhelming you with the flavour.

If this description sounds useful to you and you are willing to shell out for an excellent tea, then this is the best choice for you.

However, if you are a lover of bold flavours, you might want to go for broken tea leaves. Now, just because the tea leaves are broken, it does not automatically indicate that you got the lowest quality there is. Remember, there are the fanning and the dust in tea bags to claim the "lowest quality" label. As for broken tea leaves, some of them will still contain the tips that make your tea experience sweeter. Also, broken tea leaves steep faster. This is an excellent choice for you if you are not the type who likes to wait a little longer.

WHAT ARE THE TEA BENEFITS YOU ARE AFTER?

Now that we are done with the technicalities, we proceed to the personal part. What are the benefits of the tea you are after? Would you like to get slimmer? Would you want to keep your system clean? Do you have problems with your metabolism and your daily bowel movement? Would you like to avoid cancer and other deadly diseases?

Do you want to stay calm or focused?

It depends on what you want and what your body needs. Of course, you should consider what your body needs first, and if you think that it has already improved or have reached the state that you want, you may move on to *what you truly want.*

Below is a list that contains the many benefits of some of the best tea that you can use for tea cleansing. While all the teas promote weight loss, some of them are more effective. Feel free to check the list and get the tea that gives you the most beneficial effects.

TEA	BENEFITS
Black Tea	- reduces the risk for atherosclerosis
- reduces the risks for kidney stones
- prevents osteoporosis
- helps with weight loss
- helps cure intestinal disorders
- helps relieve asthma
- balances the blood pressure
- helps prevent cancer
- helps maintain your oral health
- gets rid of toxins in the body
- gives focus and mental alertness
- helps prevent heart disease
Chamomile (Tisanes)	- gets rid of diarrhea
- helps alleviate anxiety
- helps alleviate mouth swelling

Dandelion (Tisanes)	• helps cure a hangover
	• has antimicrobial properties
	• helps alleviate premenstrual symptoms
	• lowers high cholesterol levels
	• helps relieve gastrointestinal issues
	• helps manage diabetes
	• helps manage hypertension
	• boosts the function of liver and kidneys
Ginger (Tisanes)	• gets rid of nausea
	• helps alleviate morning sickness
	• gets rid of dizziness
	• helps relieve menstrual pain
Ginseng	• lowers high blood sugar levels
	• balances the blood pressure
	• enhances mental function
	• cures erectile dysfunction

| Green Tea | - helps with weight loss
- boosts your metabolism
- reduces high cholesterol levels
- gives focus and mental alertness
- oral leukoplakia
- cervical dysplasia
- balances the blood pressure
- prevents osteoporosis |
|---|---|
| Oolong Tea | - provides focus and mental alertness
- helps with weight loss
- boosts metabolism
- encourages healthy skin
- helps keep your bones healthy
- helps prevent cancer
- helps relieve stress |

Peppermint (Tisanes)	- helps alleviate stomach pain
- gets rid of bloatedness
- helps relieve stress
- strengthens immune system
- helps with weight loss
- helps relieve asthma
- prevents halitosis or bad breath
- relieves muscle pain and fatigue
- helps relieve chest congestion
- helps cure migraine, nausea, and vomiting
Pu-Erh Tea	- gives focus and mental alertness
- prevents atherosclerosis
- helps with weight loss
- helps prevent cancer
- has anti-aging properties
- has anti-radiation properties
- protects your dental health
- protects the lining of stomach

| White Tea | - helps with weight loss
- has antibacterial and antiviral properties
- helps in managing diabetes
- helps maintain reproductive health in good condition
- helps prevent cancer
- has anti-aging properties
- reduces risk of cardiovascular disease
- protects the skin from UV rays |
|---|---|

If you do not like tea cleansing with true teas, of course, you are free to choose any from the tisanes. Just do not veer away from your choices between true teas and tisanes. Never opt for commercialized slimming or dieting teas as you are not sure what other chemicals they contain. They are already too processed to claim to be natural.

There are other tisanes or herbal tea that are also good for tea cleansing such as milk thistle tea, cayenne pepper tea, burdock tea, red clover tea, hibiscus tea, garlic tea, cilantro tea, and chicory tea. In fact, there is a whole lot of choices for you out there; they may be true teas, or tisanes (herbal), it merely depends on the benefits that you want.

Chapter 9: Cleansing Plan

Now that we have, pretty much, everything in place, let us now move on to your tea cleansing plan. Again, let me remind you that you should never starve yourself, it's not such a good idea, plus it defeats the purpose of taking in tea that will improve your metabolism.

Remember, having too much of anything is wrong. Having none is just as bad.

However, there are ones that you need to avoid or lessen the consumption of for the cleansing plan to take effect properly. Here they are:

- cigarettes or tobacco
- alcohol
- coffee
- sugar
- honey
- artificial sweeteners

Lessen the consumption of:

- dairy products

You may also have your true teas decaffeinated if you find them a little too bold for you or if it prevents you from having a good night's sleep.

Feel free to enjoy:

- any fresh fruit

- any fresh vegetables

- raw unsalted almonds, walnuts, macadamias, and cashews

- legumes – can be dried or canned, such as kidney beans, chickpeas, lentils

- lean red meat, chicken (without the skin).

- Eggs: preferably organic

- Olive oil (preferably extra virgin), Coconut oil (unprocessed)

- Seeds: raw unsalted sesame, pumpkin, and

- sunflower seeds
- Water: from one to three liters of water per day
- Fish: fresh, canned in water or olive oil

A few tea cleansing recipes to help you through your day are,

- Green Tea Cleansing Drink
- Cleansing Dandelion Tea
- Fresh Cranberry Juice
- Fruit mix drink
- Strawberry Banana Yogurt Smoothie
- Cherry Chocolate Milk Smoothie
- Blue Rose Cucumber Smoothie
- Kale and Celery Smoothie

Surely, with all the information here, you should be able to start your cleansing tea diet. Make sure you follow them as much as possible. Tea cleansing will help you shed a few pounds, of course, it depends on how religious you will be on sticking to your plans.

Take advantage of the fact that tea stores are available near you. You can, pretty much, find tea anywhere. You can even order them online. If there is anything that you should be doing right now, that would be re-examining yourself and finding out which tea will give you the benefits you need. Start the healthy routine as soon as you can.

Chapter 10: Reminders and Take-Aways

Now that we have reached the end of the book, it would be nice to leave you some parting reminders and takeaways, so here goes:

- As for your metabolism, since you are just about to start your tea cleansing, you need not worry about how messed up your metabolism is. You are not the only one who is having a hard time with it. It will soon get sorted out, and once it does, you can start trying other teas to experience their benefits.

- Tea cleansing is also meant to help calm your mind so you can quickly focus on the things that needed your utmost attention. It also naturally enhances your metabolism, regardless of your age. You know it is true how metabolism slows down as we age, and some of us even start thinking as if there is no way they can fix it anymore. In fact, you can adjust the metabolism issue with just warm water every morning, around 30 minutes after you wake up. However, adding tea to it just makes it more fun, flavourful, the effects are even faster, plus you are showered with more benefits than only one. So, why stick to only plain water, right?

- You may also try performing some meditation for 15 minutes every day. The benefits of your tea consumption, such as better focus, will be enhanced by doing the meditation.

- When eating, feel free also to try your best to cut down, if not avoid altogether, the dressings. I understand, they make the salad less bland, but they are not as healthy as they seem.

- Salads contain enzymes that help your digestion. Enzymes work by breaking down molecules, in this case, your fat molecules. That means you are taking in food and drinks that all focus on keeping you healthy and trim. The effects of what you eat complement each other, so do not be surprised if you start seeing the results in a week or two. Trust me; tea is one of the few things that exist that shows fast results.

- I know I have mentioned this earlier already, but

repeating it just for the sake of gently reminding you would not hurt. So, remember to watch the portioning of what you eat. If you love chocolates, eat a portion of it, wait for about 20 minutes, then drink your favourite tea. That way, the tea makes sure that nothing sticks or gets stuck in your digestive tract. The same thing applies to everything else that you like to eat. Portioning and then tea drinking.

- True tea has steeping guides because they are a bit too sensitive, especially if you opt to buy the more exceptional lot. Tisanes have steeping time as well, but really, it depends on how much flavour you want from the herbal tea. They are not as sensitive as true tea.

- Also, never drink tea on an empty stomach. It might prove to be a little too harsh for an empty stomach, even if your tea of choice is meant to protect your stomach's lining. **Always remember: Eat first, wait for 20 minutes, then drink your tea.** You know, that 20-minute rule is not weird. It does not exist for tea only. In fact, that is how it should be even if you are just drinking plain, room temperature water. The 20-minute rule does magic with your metabolism.

- Add lemon to your tea if you think the flavour is a little too bold for you. Lemon will make it taste lighter, with a spike. If you have cinnamon, you can try adding that to your tea instead of lemon. Apart from discovering new flavours by adding them to your tea, you also get the benefits that they offer.

- There are teas that curbs hunger and cravings. So, in case your cravings suddenly attack at an ungodly hour, drink that hunger-curbing tea instead. You will not only prevent yourself from snacking mindlessly in the middle of the night, but you will also have a better sleep.

- Tea cleansing does not only clean your gut and the rest of your system, but it also gets rid of the negative energy around you. It makes you feel refreshed, and lighter. It naturally enhances your mood and makes you a calmer. If you choose the right kind of tea, it can help you go to sleep, focus, or just calm down. Do not restrict yourself with only a little information. Feel free to read more about teas. It is such a marvel to discover how beneficial these seemingly very simple drinks are.

- If you enjoy your tea in teabags, do not throw the tea bags after one brew. You can still brew them for the second time. However, the tea will be a bit weaker by then. Again, it is your choice if you will drink the tea, or just place the used bag in the freezer. That used tea bag does wonders for puffy eyes and even acne. Now, you see how excellent tea is? It cleans you from the inside out.

- So, you want something sweet that does not taste like tea, but you are not doing anything about it because you know you will soon feel guilty? Fret no more. You may enjoy hot chocolate, from cocoa tablea. It is best experienced when appropriately crushed. And you will not feel guilty because it is, pretty much, as good as the tea. It is also packed with anti-oxidants. Feel free to enjoy it from time to time when you are craving for coffee or something else other than tea.

- If you want to enjoy your tea cold, steep it in hot or warm water first. You may follow the guide for steeping true teas using the recommended temperature of water. Once appropriately steeped, you may transfer it to a glass and let it cool for a bit. Add ice and enjoy.

There are different ways and tastes of every tea, and whatever suits you best is your choice. A person is not restricted to one kind of tea. I only suggest that you address what ails you first because that is the most sensible thing to do. Something that ails you is not something that can afford to wait, or you risk aggravating it. Once you are done with whatever it is that ails you, then you can try the other flavours for fun, for their benefits, or for flavour hunting.

right kind of tea, it can help you go to sleep, focus, or just calm down. Do not restrict yourself with only a little information. Feel free to read more about teas. It is such a marvel to discover how beneficial these seemingly very simple drinks are.

- If you enjoy your tea in teabags, do not throw the tea bags after one brew. You can still brew them for the second time. However, the tea will be a bit weaker by then. Again, it is your choice if you will drink the tea, or just place the used bag in the freezer. That used tea bag does wonders for puffy eyes and even acne. Now, you see how excellent tea is? It cleans you from the inside out.

- So, you want something sweet that does not taste like tea, but you are not doing anything about it because you know you will soon feel guilty? Fret no more. You may enjoy hot chocolate, from cocoa tablea. It is best experienced when appropriately crushed. And you will not feel guilty because it is, pretty much, as good as the tea. It is also packed with anti-oxidants. Feel free to enjoy it from time to time when you are craving for coffee or something else other than tea.

- If you want to enjoy your tea cold, steep it in hot or warm water first. You may follow the guide for steeping true teas using the recommended temperature of water. Once appropriately steeped, you may transfer it to a glass and let it cool for a bit. Add ice and enjoy.

There are different ways and tastes of every tea, and whatever suits you best is your choice. A person is not restricted to one kind of tea. I only suggest that you address what ails you first because that is the most sensible thing to do. Something that ails you is not something that can afford to wait, or you risk aggravating it. Once you are done with whatever it is that ails you, then you can try the other flavours for fun, for their benefits, or for flavour hunting.

Conclusion

Check your journal and imprint a week where you have a total separation from capacities or occasions that may crash your cleansing diet, for example, weddings, birthdays or unique event suppers. A few people may encounter a "purging" response in the initial few days of cleanse, including headaches or loose bowel movements. This is because of the sudden withdrawal of specific nourishments, notwithstanding incitement of cleansing your organs. These indications inevitably die down in 24 to 48 hours.

THE CLEANSING TEA is not at all like another eating regimen arranges out there furnishes you with a small trick sheet to re-wiring your whole framework for fruitful weight reduction. Rather than starving yourself and subjecting your body to extreme changes in schedule, this gives a perfect structure to permit your body a move to return to such a framework, to the point that it begins performing better through and through and gives you the abundantly necessary change that you needed to find in your self-perception.

However, the advantages do not merely end here. The body reset arrangement enhances your resting, eating designs and for the most part just aides the body control itself. Undertaking this eating regimen arrangement may appear like very much an undertaking however at last as the idiom goes, the verification is in the pudding! Once you begin getting results, it will make you feel a great deal more sure about own self and the viability of this eating routine!

Final Words

Thank you again for purchasing this book! I really hope this book is able to help you.

The next step is for you to **join our email newsletter** to receive updates on any upcoming new book releases or promotions. You can sign-up for free and as a bonus, you will also receive our "*7 Fitness Mistakes You Don't Know You're Making*" book! This bonus book breaks down many of the most common fitness mistakes and will demystify many of the complexities and science of getting into shape. Having all this fitness knowledge and science organized into an actionable step-by-step book will help you get started in the right direction in your fitness journey! To join our free email newsletter and grab your free book. Please visit the link and signup: **www.hmwpublishing.com/gift**

Finally, if you enjoyed this book, then I would like to ask you for a favor, would you be kind enough to leave a review for this book? It would be greatly appreciated!

Thank you and good luck in your journey!

Sugar Detox

The Ultimate Beginner's Diet Guide Recipes Solution To Sugar Detox Your Body & Quickly Beat the Sugar Cravings Addiction Naturally

By *Simone Jacobs*

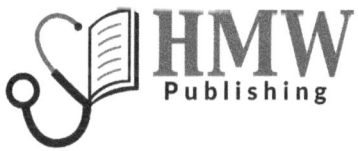

For more great books visit:

HMWPublishing.com

Table of Contents

Introduction...........................11

Chapter 1: Sugar – The Root of All Health Evil 13

What is Sugar? 15

The Six (6) Kinds of Sugar...............15

Blame It on Fructose.......................16

Sugar Addiction: A Not So Sweet Love Story 17

How Does Sugar Destroy Us? Let Us Count the Ways................................19

Bad for Your Teeth..........................19

Cause Liver Problems 19

Cause Insulin Resistance and Diabetes 20

Cause Cancer...................................21

Excessive Weight Gain and Obesity 21

Raises Cholesterol Level 22

Chapter 2: Why You Need to End Your Love Affair with Sugar 25

The Benefits of Sugar Detoxification 25

Regulate Insulin Production............ 25

Improve the Insulin Sensitivity 25

Normalizes Cortisol Production 26

Lowers the Production of Ghrelin, the Hunger Hormone 27

Cures and Prevent Leptin Resistance 28

Improves the Effects of Peptide YY or PPY 29

Naturally Increases the Levels of Dopamine 29

Resets Tastes Buds 30

Reduce Inflammation 30

Boosts Detoxification 32

Food You Need to Avoid 32

Sugar 32

Grains and Gluten 33

Factory-Made and Processed Foods 35

Alcohol 38

Caffeine 38

Starting Your Sugar Detoxification: 39

What Foods to Eat 39

Exercise 47

Supplements 48

Hydrate 49

Write Your Experience 49

Unwind and Relax 50

Get Into the Rhythm 51

Get Enough Sleep 52

Chapter 3: Preparing for Sugar Detox 54

Sugar Detox Your Kitchen 54

Supply Your Kitchen with the Good Stuff 56

Groceries 56

Detoxifying Bath Supplies 59

Sugar Detox Journal 60

Supplements 60

Testing Tools to Monitor Your Progress 64

Exercise Clothing 65

Water Filter and Bottle 65

Reduce Consumption of Sugar, Caffeine, and Alcohol 66

How Do I Deal with Detox Symptoms 67

Set Your Mind 73

Measure Your Progress.................... 76

Weight... 76

Height.. 76

Waist Size 77

Hip Size 77

Thigh Circumference 77

Blood Pressure 77

Chapter 4: What to Expect and How to Get Through 78

Day 3: This Is It! 78

Day 4: Ten More Days to Go! 79

Day 5: I made it Through! 79

Day 6: Almost Half Way Done! 79

Day 7: One Week Down! 80

Day 8: One More Week! 80

Day 9: Yeah! I Am Feeling Good! No More Cravings! 81

Day 10: I Feel A Bit Weak, But This Is Not As Hard As I Thought. I Should Continue Eating Healthy! 82

Day 11: I Sleep Like a Baby, But I Am Craving For Something Sweet 82

Day 12: Am I Losing Any Weight? The Two Weeks Are Almost Up. 83

Day 13: Almost Done! What Do I Do After? 84

Day 14: I Made It! 85

Your Daily Ritual 85

Morning 85

Afternoon 86

Evening 86

Chapter 5: Sugar Detox Meal Plan Sample 88

Shopping List 94

Chapter 6: Sugar Detox Recipes 98

Spinach and Cheese Baked Eggs 98

Toasted Tamari Almond Snack 100

Sweet Pepper Cheesy Poppers 102

Baked Stuffed Chicken &Spinach Recipe 104

Feta and Cucumber Relish 106

Feta and Sun-Dried Tomato Frittata 108

Spinach Cheesy 111

Asian Turkey Lettuce Cups 113

Peanut Butter Smoothie 115

Fresh Herb Marinated Grilled Chicken 117

Vegetable Soup 118

Vanilla-Flavored Chia Pudding 122

Mini Frittatas..................124

Chicken and Cilantro Salad............127

Bean and Chicken Stew...................129

Mini Cheesy Zucchini Bites............132

Mediterranean-Inspired Spicy Feta Dip 134

Cheesy Cauliflower Bread Sticks.....136

Italian-Inspired Green Bean Salad..139

Egg Muffin...................142

Lemon-Garlic Chicken Drumsticks.144

Zucchini Salad...................147

Homemade Salsa...................149

Final Words 151

INTRODUCTION

This book contains proven steps and strategies on how you can successfully overcome your sugar addiction. This Sugar Detox guide will help you discover how you can still eat delicious meals and become healthier.

Moreover, you'll learn the advantages of kicking junk, sugary and processed foods out of your life. Likewise, will also explain and reveal how to deal with the symptoms of sugar detox. Lastly, this book will also provide you with delicious meal plans, action plan, and Sugar Detox-friendly recipes to help you get started right away!

Also, before you get started, I recommend you joining our email newsletter to receive updates on any upcoming new book releases or promotions. You can sign-up for free, and as a bonus, you will receive a free gift. Our "*Health & Fitness Mistakes You Don't Know You're Making*" book! This book has been written to demystify, expose the top do's and don'ts and to finally equip you with the information you need to get in the best shape of your life. Due to the overwhelming amount of mis-information and lies told by magazines and self-proclaimed "gurus", it's becoming harder and harder to get reliable information to get in shape. As opposed to having to go through dozens of biased, unreliable and untrustworthy sources to get your health & fitness information. Everything you need to help you has been broken down in this book for you to easily follow and to immediately get results to achieve your desired fitness goals in the shortest amount of time.

Once again, to join our free email newsletter and to receive a free copy of this valuable book, please visit the link and signup now: www.hmwpublishing.com/gift

Chapter 1: Sugar – The Root of All Health Evil

Oh, sugar! How do I love thee? Let me count the ways. Studies reveal that the average American consumes about 22.7 teaspoons of sugar daily. Even without adding sugar to your food, you are eating processed foods that are packed with sugar to enhance the flavor and texture of the food and to act as a preservative to extend its shelf life.

To give you a picture, here are the most common food you consume every day and their sugar content:

Food	Size	Amount of sugar (1 teaspoon = 4.2 grams)
Ketchup	3 tablespoons	1.77 teaspoons
Oreo cookies	3 cookies	2.49 teaspoons
Low-fat fruit yogurt	8 ounces	6.16 teaspoons
Cola	12 ounces	7.93 teaspoons

Lucky charms	1 cup	2.55 teaspoons
Wheat bread	2 slices	0.66 teaspoons
Pork and beef bologna	4 slices	1.18 teaspoons

The natural foods you eat also contain natural sugar. For example, 27 grams of corn, 1, 135 cups of rice, 454 eggs, and 7 red apples contain 22.7 teaspoons of sugar.

If you are not mindful of what you eat, you can easily consume excessive amounts of sugar than what your body needs. **According to the American Heart Association (AHA), men need 9 teaspoons or 37.5 grams of sugar and women need 6 teaspoons or 25 grams of sugar daily. f**

Our bodies need sugar or glucose to function. To understand the importance of sugar, let's take a quick look at what sugar is and in what forms we need to make it for the best benefits, specifically glucose and fructose.

What is Sugar?

Sugar is a pure form of carbohydrate that comes in many ways.

The Six (6) Kinds of Sugar

- Glucose – occurs naturally in plant juices and fruits. This pure sugar can be carried in the blood. It is the other half of the sucrose or table sugar, paired with fructose.

- Fructose - occurs naturally in cane sugar, fruits, honey, and root vegetables. It is the other half of sucrose, paired with glucose.

- Galactose – combines with glucose to form lactose. This is also known as milk sugar, and it makes up 5 percent of cow's milk.

- Sucrose – or commonly known as table sugar. This sugar naturally occurs in sugar cane and beets.

- Maltose - made up of two joined glucose molecules.

- High fructose corn syrup – this sugar is chemically

very similar to sucrose. However, half of the glucose is converted to fructose.

All carbohydrates, once consumed, are converted into glucose during digestion, which is the sugar that our body needs.

The problem is we consume food with too added sugar. We add table sugar in almost every food we eat – from coffee, tea, baked goods, and more. Table sugar is composed of 50 percent glucose and 50 percent fructose.

Glucose, as mentioned before, is metabolized throughout the body – the glucose is absorbed from the intestines into the bloodstream and then distributed to all the cells of the body. Glucose is vital to the proper functioning of the brain since it is the primary source of fuel of the billions of neural nerve cells in the brain. Neurons can't store glucose themselves, so they need a constant supply from the bloodstream.

Blame It on Fructose

Fructose is processed mainly by the liver and is turned

into fat, which can build up and enter the bloodstream. Moreover, the market is also flooded with products – from soda to soup, with high fructose corn syrup. High fructose corn syrup is cheaper and sweeter than sucrose made from sugar cane and beets. What's the difference? Not enough to fuss about since they both contain fructose and everyone can benefit from eating less, if not eliminating it, from their diet.

When you consume too much fructose, it causes various health risks, including type 2 diabetes, insulin resistance, hypertension, and obesity. In fact, nephrologist Richard Johnson from the University of Colorado Denver, states that when you trace the path of the illness back to its primary cause, you will find your way again to sugar, fructose in particular.

Sugar Addiction: A Not So Sweet Love Story

If an extra slice of cake or chocolate has tempted you, then you know exactly how addictive sweets are and how difficult it is to cut back. To put it just, sugar in our bloodstream stimulates the same pleasure centers in the brain that responds to cocaine and heroin.

Sugar is not all bad for us. In fact, our body needs sugar. Johnson theorized that our ancestors evolved to become an efficient processor of fructose for survival, storing even the smallest amounts it as fat during times when food is abundant for use during the scarce seasons. Thus, today, we have a craving for fruit sugar.

For some people, sugar can end up in a full-blown addiction, the same way someone is addicted to abuse drugs like cannabis, amphetamine, and nicotine. There is no difference. The only dissimilarity is that sugar is legal and is not a controlled substance. In fact, people who are addicted to alcohol and drugs claim that craving for junk and sweet foods is similar. The worst part, sugar is not a regulated product. Often, we consume sugary foods without knowing the risks that it poses to our health.

How Does Sugar Destroy Us? Let Us Count the Ways.

Sugar is a bad habit, and it's a bad habit that's hard to break. Most of the time, we don't realize that overeating sweets and junk food are not a problem. To give you an idea just how bad sugar is for your health, here are some of their long-term effects.

Bad for Your Teeth

Added sugar, high fructose corn syrup, and sucrose contain calories without any essential nutrients. Hence, they are called empty calories – they contain no essential fats, vitamins, minerals, or protein – just pure energy.

When you get 10 to 20 percent or more of your calories from sugar, this can cause nutrient deficiency and health problems.

Sugar is also bad for the teeth because it is a source of digestible energy for the harmful bacteria in the mouth.

Cause Liver Problems

As mentioned earlier, sugar is broken down into two simple sugars, fructose, and glucose. We need glucose in our body while there is no physiological need for fructose. Moreover, fructose can only be metabolized in the liver, where it is transformed into glycogen and stored in the liver when not used.

It is not a problem if you only eat small amounts of fructose from fruits and you are physically active. However, if you overeat fructose-rich food, you will overload your liver, forcing it to turn the fructose into fat. When you repeatedly eat a significant amount of sugar, it can lead to a non-alcoholic fatty liver and cause various health problems.

Keep in mind that it is almost impossible to overeat fructose from eating fruits since they contain very little fructose. The problem starts when you consume foods with too much sugar additives.

Cause Insulin Resistance and Diabetes

Insulin is a hormone that is vital to various bodily functions. It helps blood sugar or glucose to enter the cells from the bloodstream. It also tells the cells when to begin burning glucose instead of fat.

When you have high levels of glucose, the body works

overtime to produce insulin, flooding the cells with the hormone. Thus, the cells become resistant to it. When you are insulin resistant, it leads to various diseases, including obesity, metabolic syndrome, cardiovascular disease, and especially type II diabetes.

Cause Cancer

Insulin does not only regulate the glucose levels in the body. It also controls the growth and multiplication of cells, which is the characteristic of cancer.

Many scientists believe that if you consume too much sugar, the constant high levels of insulin in the body can cause cancer.

Excessive Weight Gain and Obesity

Not only is fructose metabolized differently from glucose. Studies also show that fructose does not have the same satiety as glucose. People who drank fructose-sweetened beverage felt hungrier and less satiated than people who drank glucose-sweetened drink. Furthermore, the fructose does not lower ghrelin, a hunger hormone, as efficiently as glucose can.

Over time, because fructose isn't as filling, you will feel

the need to increase your caloric intake, eating more food, which, in turn, causes weight gain.

Many studies reveal that sugar is the main cause childhood obesity. Kids who drink sugar-sweetened beverages are 60 percent more at risk of obesity. If you want to lose weight, the most important thing you can do is to reduce sugar consumption.

Raises Cholesterol Level

For a long time, people blamed saturated fat for heart disease, which is the number one cause of death in the world. Recent studies reveal that saturated fat is not to blame. Evidence suggests that SUGAR and not fat, is the leading cause of heart disease, due to the harmful effects of metabolizing fructose.

Studies reveal that high amounts of fructose raise the triglycerides, dense, small low-density lipoprotein and oxidized LDL, increase the levels of glucose in the blood, insulin levels, and abdominal obesity in as short as 10 weeks.

Consequently, various observational studies reveal a healthy relationship between high sugar consumption and the risk of heart disease.

Aside from the chronic diseases, most of the people who are addicted to sugar experience the following symptoms:

- Heart rate changes
- Mood changes
- Vision changes
- Seizures and convulsions
- Diarrhea
- Poor equilibrium/dizziness
- Weakness and fatigue
- Rash/hives
- Joint pain
- Memory loss
- Headaches and migraines
- Vomiting and nausea
- Insomnia/sleep problems

- Weight-loss problems

With all the health problems that can be traced back to our love for sweet foods, there is a need to detoxify from sugar. Our bodies have evolved to get by with just the smallest amount of fructose. The problem is that our world is flooded with high fructose corn syrup and sucrose. It can be challenging to break up with sugar, but it is an effort that we need to do for our overall health.

Chapter 2: Why You Need to End Your Love Affair with Sugar

Now that you understand how too much sugar and sugar addiction can be detrimental to your health, it is time for detoxification and rehabilitation. It will take considerable effort and willpower to reset your body from a state of chaos. However, rebooting your system will benefit you in the long run.

The Benefits of Sugar Detoxification

Regulate Insulin Production

Mentioned earlier, too much sugar increases the production of insulin, which can often cause insulin resistance and lead to diabetes. Too much fructose also turns into stored fat. When you detoxify, the output of insulin in your body normalizes, which reduces the storage of fat in the belly and food cravings.

Improve the Insulin Sensitivity

When the body has high levels of insulin all the time, the

cells become resistant to it. Thus, the body is unable to regulate blood sugar levels efficiently. Rebooting your system allows the body to adjust the production of insulin, which improves blood sugar regulation, helping you lose weight and improve your health.

Normalizes Cortisol Production

Cortisol is a hormone produced by the adrenal glands and the levels of the cortisol in the body rise and fall during different times during the whole day. It is at its highest level in the morning to help you get ready and move at the start the day, and it is at its lowest at night to help you wind down for a good night's rest. When your body has too much blood sugar, it weakens the adrenal glands, which affects cortisol production, a hormone that also helps regulate the blood sugar on a metabolic level.

When the adrenal glands are tired, it is unable to produce the right amount of cortisol that you need in a day. Hence, you will feel sluggish and low in energy. Instinctively, you will want to reach for a quick fix and most of the time. You will munch on a carbohydrate snack, coke, sugary food, or coffee. This is only a temporary solution, one that leads to a spike in blood sugar and insulin production, which later ends up with your blood sugar crashing and ultimately, weakening your adrenal glands even more. The result is a continuous low cortisol production, which is evident in the morning when you wake up feeling tired and unrested even after a night's sleep.

When you detoxify, the system resets, helping your adrenal glands recover and enable it to supply your body with the right amounts of cortisol at different times of the day.

Lowers the Production of Ghrelin, the Hunger Hormone

When you consume sugary food, your body increases its production of insulin so that the sugar can be converted and used by the cells of your body. It also increases the levels of leptin, a hormone that regulates fat storage and appetite, which decreases the production of ghrelin, controlling your food intake. The idea is that when you eat, your body automatically works to let you know that you should feel less hungry.

The problem occurs when you consume too much fructose. The cycle that should tell you that you are full does not happen. You already know that the body uses glucose. Glucose also suppresses the production of ghrelin and stimulates the production of leptin, which both works to suppress the appetite.

Fructose, on the other hand, not only affects the regulation of ghrelin, but it also interferes with the brain's communication with leptin, which leads to overeating. This is why fructose leads to excessive weight gain, insulin resistance, metabolic syndrome, and increased belly fat, as well as the long list of chronic diseases.

When you limit your fructose to healthy levels, it regulates and lowers the production of the hunger hormone ghrelin.

Cures and Prevent Leptin Resistance

Research reveals that when you consume fructose, you generate more fat in your liver compared to other types of sugar. Moreover, fructose blocks the body's ability to burn fat.

When you eat fewer calories, but you eat large amounts of fructose or your diet is high in sugar it will still cause a fatty liver, insulin resistance, and leptin resistance.

You have learned earlier that when you eat sugar the leptin levels of rising and signal your body that it is full so that you will stop eating. However, when you are leptin resistant, your body no longer responds to leptin. You end up eating more because you don't feel full or satiated. Hence, sugar detoxification will significantly benefit you.

Improves the Effects of Peptide YY or PPY

Peptide YY is a hormone released in the intestines and colon that controls appetite. When the sugar level in your body is unstable of high, it impairs the effects of PYY in appetite suppression.

Naturally Increases the Levels of Dopamine

Sugary and junk food changes the brain's chemistry, making you want more and more of them, even when you are full. Dr. Robert H. Lustig, pediatric endocrinologist, and Dr. Elissa S. Epel, a psychologist, explain that when you consume large amounts of sugar, your brain releases massive amounts of dopamine, the hormone responsible for making you feel good. When there is a surge of dopamine, it causes the dopamine receptors to down-regulate.Meaning, there are now fewer receptors for them, so the next time you eat sugary and junk foods, their "feel-good" effect is blunted, thus, you need to eat more of them to get the same feeling of reward.

Sugar detoxification resets the reward pathways of the brain, allowing you to feel pleasure from eating real food.

Resets Tastes Buds

According to research at the Monell Chemical Senses Center, which was published in the American Journal of Clinical Nutrition, avoiding or eliminating sugar for a period will reboot your taste buds. When you consume low amounts of sugar for a couple of months, even foods with little sugar will taste sweet. This means that when you detoxify, you will be able to enjoy delicious treats more, you will be quickly satisfied with a smaller amount, and you will be less likely to overeat.

Reduce Inflammation

If you can recall your biology lesson about inflammation, you will remember that our bodies depend on temporary swelling to help fight infections and injuries – the inflammation cleans cellular debris, kill pathogens, and create protection to help to heal. Inflammation of a wound is a symptom that indicates the body has it is doing its job, the swelling, redness, slight tenderness, and warm feeling is the body's defense at work.

However, when the inflammatory response is turned on all the time? When you experience chronic inflammation, the immune system attacks normal cells by mistake, and the process that normally helps the body heals causes destruction.

Dave Grotto, RD, a spokesperson for the American Dietetic Association says the sugar cause inflammatory disease. When the body is unable to regulate the sugar and insulin levels in the body, a hidden inflammation in the body can cause chronic infections. When the blood sugar is high, the body generates more free radicals that damage the cells of the body, stimulating a response from the immune system, which causes inflammation that you cannot see.

Eliminating sugar, processed foods, and ordinary food sensitives, together with consuming foods that help fight off inflammation, reduce your risk of developing chronic diseases.

Boosts Detoxification

As mentioned in the previous benefit, too much sugar in the body increases free radicals. When you detoxify, you not only reduce the damage to your cells caused by free radicals, you also help your body get rid of other toxins that make you fat.

The benefits you get from detoxifying from sugar, as well as processed food, will help your body heal. When you avoid sugar, you will not only lose weight, but you will also benefit from the long-term health improvements.

Food You Need to Avoid

That is the question. To get the full benefit of sugar detoxification, you will not only need to avoid sugar. You will also need to avoid other types of food.

Sugar

By this point, you probably know why you need to cut back on sugar. However, it can be a scary change, especially if you have a sweet tooth. Don't worry; you won't go crazy during your detoxification. Even the most stubborn cravings and addictions will be curved. People who already detoxed claim the incredible change in as little as 24 hours and their desires have lessened

Grains and Gluten

Gluten is the two most common food sensitivities. Most people do not realize that they are sensitive to certain foods because this condition is not a real allergy like shellfish or peanut allergy, which creates hives, close the throat, swell the tongues, and can kill the person within minutes.

Unlike true allergies, food sensitivity is a subtle reaction to food. It is hidden because the small changes usually occur in the digestive tract. When you have food sensitivities, the lining in the gastrointestinal tract, particularly the intestine gradually becomes damaged and porous, a condition called a leaky gut, wherein food particles enter the bloodstream, creating a response to the body's immune system.

Earlier, I have mentioned about how the body protects itself and inflammation is a good sign that the body's defences are working. However, when you have a leaky gut, your body is consistently in a state of low-grade inflammation as a reaction to the foreign particles in your bloodstream, resulting in many various symptoms that you would not connect to the food you eat. Some of these symptoms include brain fog, fatigue, depression, headaches, sinus problems, allergies, reflux, irritable bowel, autoimmune disease, joint pain, and skin diseases, such as eczema and acne.

Moreover, low-grade inflammation also triggers insulin resistance, which causes weight gain.

Gluten, a protein found in oats, spelled, rye, barley, and wheat. Some people are unable to digest it, causing a leaky gut. Additionally, because of genetic modification, a new strain of wheat has been created. This grain contains amylopectin A, a super-starch that triggers spikes in blood sugar. Two slices of bread made from this new corn raise the blood sugar more than 2 tablespoons of table sugar.

Gluten sensitivity, together with super-starch, triggers more inflammation, which increases the risk of diabetes and obesity.

All grains, including cereals, bread, and snacks, even the

gluten-free kind, can spike blood sugar and insulin because they contain carbohydrates.

Moreover, research shows that when you eat high carb food, mainly if you have been consuming high-fructose food and your liver has been metabolizing fructose for quite some time, even when there is no fructose in your diet, your liver will convert the glucose, found in flour and bread, into fructose. Hence, during your detox, as mentioned earlier, you will need to avoid high carb food, such as rice, bread, and another non-vegetable carbohydrate.

Factory-Made and Processed Foods

As you already know, these foods are packed with artificial sweeteners and high-fructose corn syrup. They also made with preservatives, chemicals, additives, monosodium glutamate or MSG, and hydrogenated fats. MSG cause insulin spike, leading to cravings, hunger, and overeating.

During your detox, eat only food that is low-glycemic, contain good fats, proteins, phytonutrients, fiber, minerals, and vitamins.

Keep in mind; MSG can be hidden, so watch out for these ingredients:

- Any "flavoring" or "flavors."
- Anything with "enzyme modified."
- Anything with "hydrolyzed."
- Anything containing "enzymes."
- Anything with "glutamate" in it
- Autolyzed plant protein
- Autolyzed yeast
- Barley malt
- Bouillon and broth
- Carrageenan
- Gelatin
- Glutamate
- Glutamic acid
- Hydrolyzed plant protein (HPP)

- Hydrolyzed vegetable protein (HVP)
- Malt extract
- Maltodextrin
- Natural seasonings
- Protease
- Stock
- Textured protein
- Umami
- Vegetable protein extract
- Yeast extract
- Yeast food or nutrient
- Processed and Refined Vegetable Oils

You will need to avoid sunflower, canola, soybean oil, and more. They contain omega-6 fatty acids that cause inflammation. During your detox, use extra-virgin coconut butter or extra-virgin olive oil. Extra-virgin olive oil contains polyphenols, a potent antioxidant, and anti-inflammatory compounds while coconut butter contains anti-inflammatory fats, such as lauric acid, the same fat found in breast milk. If you need oil for high-heat cooking, grape seed oil is safe.

Alcohol

Alcohol is sugar in various forms. Moreover, when you drink alcohol, it impairs self-control, so you will be most likely to overeat mindlessly. It also contains 7 calories per gram, more than the four calories per gram of sugar. It not only causes leaky gut, but it also inflames the liver.

Caffeine

Some claim that caffeine speed up metabolism in a process called thermogenesis. However, you will also get the same effect by adding spices to your dishes, such as cayenne or jalapeno pepper. Caffeine is also addictive, and when inserted into sugary drinks, you will crave for more of that food. It also increases hunger. Like sugar, caffeine causes a surge of dopamine and then it wears off eventually. Even if you do not crave for coffee, you will undoubtedly desire for more sugar.

Avoiding caffeine will reboot your system, normalize brain chemistry and lessen cravings. Even decaf contain caffeine, so it is also off limits.

Starting Your Sugar Detoxification:

What Foods to Eat

When you've removed the bad stuff, now is the time to add the proper definite replacement. All the elements of your detox help your body detoxify, shed excess weight, and heal. Avoiding the bad stuff and eating more of the excellent material optimize and accelerate your results.

Detox Pathway Boosters

To maximize your detox, you need to eat more superfoods and foods rich in phytonutrients. When your body is healthy, detoxification is smooth. When your body is toxic, especially when it's flooded with fructose, the liver gets sluggish, detox is slow, and certain toxins remain active longer than the system can handle. Hence, you get sick, and metabolism slows down. It also causes bloating, puffiness, and fluid retention.

When you are overweight, your body is high in toxins. As you lose weight during sugar detox, the toxins are released out from your fat tissues, and you will need to flush them out. Otherwise, it can impair weight loss and poison your metabolism.

Here are the foods the speed up detox:

1. Watercress
2. Wakame
3. Rosemary
4. Parsley
5. Onion
6. Lemon
7. Kombu
8. Kale
9. Ginger
10. Garlic
11. Eggs

12. Collards

13. Cilantro

14. Cayenne pepper

15. Cauliflower

16. Cabbage

17. Brussels sprouts

18. Broccoli

19. Bok Choy

20. Arame

They are rich in vitamin A and C, B vitamins, antioxidants, and phytonutrients.

Anti-Inflammatory Foods

Inflammation is your body's typical reaction to heal wounds and fight off bacteria. This is what happens when you have a sore throat, a cut, or strain. When the injury is infected, it turns, hot, red, and tender.

The inflammations that you need to be concerned about are the ones hidden inside your body and do not necessarily hurt. It's the inflammation caused by allergens, toxins, stress, bad food, the overgrowth of harmful bacteria in your gut, and low-grade infections.

Anything that causes inflammation will eventually cause insulin resistance, which produces belly fat and your body to hold on to fat cells. Earlier, I have mentioned the food that you need to avoid. Now I am going to give you the list of foods that will help minimize inflammation.

Omega 3 fatty acid-rich foods, such as:

1. Salmon
2. Eggs
3. Grass-fed beef
4. Hemp seeds
5. Chia seeds
6. Walnuts
7. Flaxseeds
8. Spices and herbs, such as turmeric
9. Berries

10. Dark-green leafy vegetables

11. Extra-virgin olive oil

12. Avocado

13. Organic poultry

14. Wild seafood

15. Non-GMO tempeh and tofu

Foods That Cure Leaky Gut and Improve Gut Function

Every individual has 500 species of bacteria in the digestive system. These bacteria help control metabolism, digestion, and inflammation. Research studies also indicate that your weight may be controlled more by that the bacteria in your gut eat than what you eat yourself.

The bacteria in your gut increase, depending on what you eat and feed them. When you eat healthy food, the right bacteria grow and help boost your metabolism. However, if you eat junk, unhealthy diet, the harmful bacteria is the once that increase. This is something you should avoid because bad bacteria produce nasty gas and toxins that cause inflammation, weight gain, puffiness, bloated belly, and diabesity or the metabolic dysfunction. This is characterized by metabolic syndrome, insulin resistance, obesity, and type 2 diabetes, which is all caused by high blood sugar and can be treated using the same treatment.

When there is an imbalance of gut bacteria in your digestive system, it damages the lining of your gut or a leaky gut, which causes inflammation, and in turn, damages metabolism, affects how the brain controls appetite, leads to insulin resistance, and of course, weight gain.

Low sugar, low starch, high fiber, and whole food diet feeds the good bacteria and starves the harmful bacteria. Foods that are rich in minerals and vitamins help improve gut function. It includes:

- Bok Choy
- Pumpkin seeds
- Kale
- Arugula
- Carrots

- Tomatoes
- Turkey
- Salmon
- Chicken
- Parsley
- Onion
- Kimchi

These foods are high in vitamin A, zinc, antioxidants, amino acids, and probiotics.

Blood Sugar Balancers

The key to balance blood sugar is protein. Each meal should contain lean, preferably organic, animal protein, paired with delicious vegetables.

If you are a vegan or a vegetarian, you may have a serious weight and health problem when you substitute meat with starchy food, such as pasta, rice, bread, and other dense carbohydrate food, when once consumed turn into sugar and lead to cravings.

Even beans and grains can be a problem since these foods spike blood sugar and insulin more than animal protein. Eating all veggies can be unhealthy unless you know what you are doing.

Yes, you need to eat less factory-farmed meat, but animal-based protein is important for most people. If they come from pasture-raised or wild sources, then animal protein can be very healthy.

Your detox will partially depend on your current metabolism and health. The sicker you are, the less room you have regarding the sugar you can consume. As you detoxify and lose weight, your resilience will increase, and after the detox period, you can experiment with beans and grains as a source of protein. However, if you currently have significant health concerns, then avoid them, for the time being.

Seeds and nuts are the exceptions when it comes to protein from plant sources. They do not spike blood sugar and are great as snacks if you do not have nut allergies. They are particularly suitable for people with diabesity since they reduce the risk of diabetes, help with weight loss, and improve metabolism since they are packed with good fats, protein, minerals, such as zinc and magnesium, and fiber, all help reverse diabesity.

Exercise

Exercise is vital during your detox period. As little as 30 minutes of moderate exercise to begin your day will jump-start your metabolism and balance your hormones, blood sugar, and brain chemistry so that you can make better food choices during the day.

Exercise regulates appetite, reduces cravings, improves insulin sensitivity, and activates detox pathways to help eliminate toxins that cause weight gain, reduce inflammation, reduce stress hormone cortisol, and encourages better help.

Exercise is the best anxiety and depression treatment. It improves self-esteem, well-being, and energy.

If you already have an exercise routine, just continue to do whatever it is you enjoy for 30 minutes. If you haven't been exercising regularly, start with a 30-minute slow or brisk walking. If you can only do 5 minutes, then start with it and do it 2 times a day. Work your way up from there. Walking is the easiest and the most accessible exercise to everyone. It doesn't require any fancy equipment or memberships. You can also try out other physical activities.

Supplements

When it comes to health and weight loss, nutrients are vital. When the body is low in essential nutrients, it craves more food, seeking to get the nutrients it needs. Hence, you end up eating more, often sugary and junk foods, searching for the nutrients that are just not there. You overeat, but the body is still starving and not satisfied.

When you start to eat more real food, you will feel more satisfied, and you will eat less. However, your body will still need the essential amount of high-quality nutrients to help your body efficiently work. Sufficient amount of vitamins and minerals are required to burn calories, regulate appetite, boost detoxification, lower inflammation, regulate cortisol or stress hormones, aid digestion, and help the cells become more sensitive to insulin.

Hydrate

Most of us are frequently dehydrated. We become even more dehydrated because most of us love to drink caffeinated drinks. Staying hydrated is one of the keys to detoxification. Fluid helps flush out environmental and metabolic toxins through the kidneys, increases energy, and improves regular bowel movements. Thus, drinking at least 8 glasses of water daily is essential during and after detox.

Studies reveal that we often mistake thirst for hunger, and eat instead of drinking. Always keep a bottle of fresh filtered water throughout the day and drink. Hydrate!

Write Your Experience

Keeping a journal and writing down your thoughts, feelings, and experiences unfiltered have been proven to reduce stress and help the process of detoxification. It's one of the best ways to stop the cycle of mindless eating. Journaling enables you to process your emotions and thoughts in a healthy, proactive way rather than just stuffing them down with bad habits and bad foods.

Writing will help you metabolize not just your thoughts,

but also your calories better. Keeping an honest account of your experience is essential. Buy a blank notebook and write about your experience every morning and at night.

Unwind and Relax

Most of us are not motivated to take a break seriously. Consider this then: when the body is stressed, it causes a spike in insulin level, increase the level of cytokines or the immune system messenger molecules that cause inflammation, and increase the level of cortisol that causes accumulation of fat on the belly.

Stress also makes you hungrier and increases your cravings for sugar and carbohydrates, which trigger metabolic dysfunction, leading to excessive weight gain. So take time unwind and take a break. The breathing exercise below will help you relax.

5-Minute Relaxation Breathing

1. Sit down as comfortably as you can – on a chair, cross-legged on a cushion on the floor, or on a propped up pillows on your bed.

2. Close your mouth and eyes.

3. Breathe slowly through your nose, counting to 5 as you inhale.

4. Hold in 5 counts.

5. Slowly exhale, counting to 5 as you breathe out.

6. Repeat for 5 minutes.

Get Into the Rhythm

Whether we like it or not, our bodies evolved into biological organisms. Whether we listen to the signals that our body is sending us or not, it follows a specific rhythm – time to sleep, wake up, eat, relax, and exercise.

Simple behavioral changes will help you get back into the rhythm, which has powerful effects, including better sleep, increased energy, weight loss, and a lot more. Thus, during your detox period, create a schedule and stick to it.

Research shows that eating very late, skipping meals, and not eating breakfast screw up your metabolism. Not eating during the day results in the night-eating syndrome or binge eating at night or getting up in the middle of the night to feed. This causes diabesity, which results in blood sugar swings.

Wake up, sleep, eat, exercise, and relax the same time every day during your detox period. You will soon notice your body getting into the rhythm. The best thing about routines is that you won't have to waste mental energy continually planning your day. Eating an early breakfast will kick-start your metabolism and allow it to burn calories all day. Likewise, you need to avoid eating 2-3 hours before bedtime to prevent fat from being stored while you sleep. While you sleep, your body grows, rebuilds, and repairs itself. However, when you are sleeping, you are burning less energy, so the last thing you want is your belly growing.

Get Enough Sleep

Not getting sufficient sleep is linked to various diseases, including obesity. Since the invention of the light bulb, humans have been staying up longer and later because we can, which disrupts the body's sync with the natural rhythm of the seasons and mess up with the first sleep pattern.

If you don't get the right amount of sleep, it increases the production of ghrelin, the hunger hormone and it decreases the production of leptin, the appetite-suppressing hormone. When it comes to sugar, sleep is a natural appetite suppressant.

If you are working night shifts, you may have noticed that you are always craving for something sweet, like ice cream, cookies, and more. Your body is not getting enough energy because you are not getting enough sleep, so you eat to get the energy your body needs.

Now that you know what you need to avoid and what you need to get more of; let's get you ready to start your sugar detox.

Chapter 3: Preparing for Sugar Detox

The key to a successful sugar detoxification is a good plan and efficient preparation. Admit it; you probably spend more time planning vacations and parties than planning how to be healthy. Before you begin your detox, design your life for success and create an environment that will automatically direct you to make healthier choices. For instance, if you have nuts instead of donuts in your pantry, then you are more likely to make a healthy decision. Set your kitchen, your mind, and your school or work environment to maximize your detox. This is Day 1 and Day 2 – the unofficial start of your sugar detox.

Sugar Detox Your Kitchen

Your kitchen is probably packed with processed, sugar-packed, and junk food. You are going to start your detox with your kitchen. Throw away any items that fall under the following categories:

1. Packaged, boxed, canned, or anything that is not real food. You can keep anything that is canned whole food, such as artichokes or sardines that contains a couple of real ingredients, such as salt or water.

2. Drinks or foods that contain any form of sugar, including artificial sweeteners, organic cane juice, maple syrup, agave, molasses, and honey, mainly any fruit juices or beverages sweetened with sugar.

3. Foods that contain refined vegetable oils, such as soybean or corn oil, and hydrogenated oil.

4. Foods with dyes, coloring, additives, preservatives, or artificial sweeteners – anything that is processed in any way and has a label.

If you are unsure if the food or drink cuts, the best thing to do is get rid of it. Be thorough!

The following items also need to go. If you don't want to throw them, transfer them somewhere that is far from your eyesight during your detox. You need to avoid them while you are detoxifying. After your detox your body, you may introduce some them back into your diet.

- Products with gluten, including, pasta, bread, bagels, etc.

- All grains, including the ones that are gluten-free.

Supply Your Kitchen with the Good Stuff

Groceries

After clearing out your cabinets and fridge, it's time to fill them with real, whole, fresh food for your detox.

Make sure you have these staples.

- Almond meal

- Anti-inflammatory and Detoxifying herbs and spices, including turmeric, thyme, cayenne pepper, rosemary, cumin, chili powder, sage, onion powder, oregano, cinnamon, cilantro, coriander, parsley, and paprika

- Apple cider vinegar

- Balsamic vinegar

- Black pepper (peppercorns that you can freshly grind)

- Broth, low-sodium (chicken or vegetable)

- Coconut butter, extra-virgin, also known as coconut oil – it may be solid or liquid at room temperature

- Coconut milk, full-fat, canned

- Dijon mustard

- Jarred or canned Kalamata olives

- Nut butter (raw if possible; choose from almond, cashew, macadamia, or walnut)

- Nuts: almonds, walnuts, macadamia pecans,

- Olive oil, extra-virgin

- Other healthy oils that you like (walnut, sesame, grapeseed, flax, or avocado)

- Sea salt

- Seeds: chia, hemp, pumpkin, flax, sesame

- Tahini or sesame seed paste—great for salad dressings and in sauces for vegetables)

- Tamari, low-sodium, gluten-free

- Unsweetened almond or hemp milk

Depending on the meal plan or the dishes, you plan to prepare for the day or the week during your detox, add the specific ingredients needed; you may not need some of the ingredients listed above. Read on through the recipes, plan your meals, and then shop for the ingredients that you need.

You may think that buying fresh, whole, good food is expensive. However, if you consider how much money you spend on takeout food, convenience food, sodas, coffee, and junk food, you would be surprised that you are spending that much money on food that is toxic. You should also consider how much you would be paying treating diseases brought on by processed and poisonous foods. When you look at the long-term benefits on your health and wallet, choosing healthy foods is way better and healthier for you.

Detoxifying Bath Supplies

Relaxing at home is easy. Lavender oil, baking soda, and Epsom salt in your bath soak will not only help you relax; the combination creates a detoxifying and relaxing routine.

For each session, you will need the following:

- 2 cups Epsom salt
- 1/2 cup baking soda
- 10 drops lavender oil

Fill the tub with water as hot as you can handle. Add the Epsom salt, baking soda, and lavender oil. To make the bathroom more relaxing, you can play some soothing music and light candles. Soak in the tub for about 20-30 minutes.

This detoxifying bath will help you de-stress and relax for

a better sleep. Your muscles and mind will benefit from this healing bath.

Sugar Detox Journal

Purchase a journal or notebook. Here you will record your experiences, thoughts, and results.

Supplements

Most people are deficient in necessary nutrients, especially people who haven't been taking care of their bodies. Before you start your detox, make sure you have the following on hand. They will supply your body with the essential nutrients that it needs. The combination is designed for long-term usage. You can find any of the supplements at your local health store.

Supplement	Dosage	Benefits

Alpha lipoic acid (ALA)	300-600 milligrams	Balances insulin and blood sugar; taken together with other supplements that optimize metabolism, blood sugar balance, and insulin.
Chromium	500-1000 micrograms	Balances insulin and blood sugar; taken together with other supplements that optimize metabolism, blood sugar balance, and insulin.
Cinnamon	500-1000 milligrams	Balances insulin and blood sugar; taken together with other supplements that optimize metabolism, blood sugar balance, and insulin.
Green tea catechins	100-200 milligrams	Balances insulin and blood sugar; taken together with other supplements that optimize metabolism, blood sugar balance, and insulin.

Magnesium citrate	200-300 milligrams (2-3 capsules) 1-2 times a day	This is used to manage constipation caused by PolyGlycopleX or PGX, mainly if your stomach is not used too much fiber. This also helps improve sleep, reduce anxiety, improve the control of blood sugar, and help cure muscle cramps.
Multivitamin and multimineral supplement	Take as indicated on the label	Help run the metabolism, improve insulin functioning, and balance blood sugar.

PolyGlycopleX or PGX (capsules or powder)	2.5-5 grams before every meal; you can take additional doses during the day to control cravings	This super fiber slows down insulin and blood sugar spikes. It also reduces needs and makes you feel full longer. Take before every meal with a large-sized glass of water. The powder form works better than the capsule. This will also help you manage night eating or night cravings. Drink the recommended eight glasses water daily to ensure the fiber moves through your body.
Purified fish oil (DHA/EPA)	2 grams	Balances blood sugar, sensitize insulin, anti-inflammatory, boosts brain function and prevents heart disease.

Vitamin D3	2,000 IU	
Zinc	15-30 milligrams	Balances insulin and blood sugar; taken together with other supplements that optimize metabolism, blood sugar balance, and insulin.

Testing Tools to Monitor Your Progress

If you have the money or if your budget allows, you may want to get the following tools that will help you test and monitor your progress.

- A glucose monitor

- A weighing scale, preferably one who uploads your weight, body composition, and BMI; if possible, one that directly uploads your info to a smartphone.

- A blood pressure monitor, if possible, one that instantly uploads your info into a smartphone

- A personal movement track to track your daily sleep and activity

Exercise Clothing

The goal here is for maximum success. You will be more likely to exercise if you keep a pair of appropriate exercise clothing and your supplies in the same place. Whenever you are ready to go, you have everything you need. Get your sneakers out of the closet or buy a new pair. Choose to clothe that you are most comfortable with. Remove any obstacles so that when you start your detox, you are ready to go.

Water Filter and Bottle

The best way to drink pure, clean water is to filter your own using a simple carbon and then pour the water into a glass or stainless steel bottle. You can find these items in the supermarket or at the home-goods store.

Reduce Consumption of Sugar, Caffeine, and Alcohol

The 2-day preparation is the start of your detox, and during this period, you will start weaning yourself off from the sugar, alcohol, and caffeine. These substances will make you feel temporarily alert and energized, but their effects wear off fast and you'll end up in a vicious crash-and-crave cycle.

- It won't be easy getting off caffeine. Do it in stages. Reduce your usual amount to half during the first day, and then reduce again by half the second day. During the official first day of your detox, go cold turkey. Take a nap if you are tired. Lots of water, a gentle exercise, a hot bath, and 1, 000 mg twice daily of vitamin C can help reduce any a headache that you may experience because of withdrawal.

- Day 2 is the time to quit alcohol and any beverage that is sweetened with artificial sweeteners or sugar. This is also the time to stop eating processed food.

How Do I Deal with Detox Symptoms

During this phase, you have already started weaning yourself from sugar and processed foods so that you may feel hungry. You will also experience the typical signs of hunger, such as a vacant sensation in the chest or abdominal area and belly growling. You will crave for sweets and feel fatigued or light-headed between meals, have trouble completing a 30-minute walk, want for coffee, experience brain fog or have difficulty concentrating, and feel anxious, moody, or short-tempered.

Rest

Relax, nap, and rest. This is vital during the first few days of detox. Rest relaxes your nervous system, the system responsible for your fight or flight response during a stressful event, helps the body repair. The first 2 days of your detox are where detoxification magic happens. Your body will adjust, and you will feel less than great, so you need to rest. This will pass once your body has transitioned.

Accept the Detox Symptoms

Feeling not so great is a great sign. It means that your

body is transitioning and eliminating the toxins from your body.

ced*Flush the Toxins*ced*

Take a detoxifying bath, get a massage, enjoy a sauna, do stretching or a gentle yoga. All these things will help reduce inflammation and increase circulation in your body, which helps reduce soreness and achiness, increase chemical secretion, move toxins, and purify the body.

Get Things Moving

Clean bowels that efficiently working prevents constipation and headaches. Here are some tips to get things moving

- Drink lots of water to flush the kidneys and clean the intestines.

- Add 2 tablespoons ground flax seeds into your soups, salads, or shakes. These are rich in fiber and absorb plenty of water.

- Take 100-150 mg of magnesium citrate twice daily will help regular bowel movement. You can take as much as 6 capsules. Stop taking or reduce the amount if the bowel becomes too loose.

- Take 1000-2000 mg vitamin C one to two times daily.

- Drink an herbal laxative, such as senna, cascara, or rhubarb before bedtime.

- Exercise helps things get moving. It's a powerful bowel stimulant and

- Sweat it out. Intense activity helps you sweat, which releases toxins through your skin. If your exercise does not cause you to sweat, take an infrared or steam sauna.

- Use an enema or suppository. There are available medications that you can buy at your local drugstore.

- Try liquid magnesium citrate. This is usually used to flush the bowel before a colonoscopy. If you can find this at your local drugstore, then you can use it. However, this solution is compelling. It can make you go in less than 4 hours, so don't leave the house and be ready.

- When all else fail, then it's time to see your doctor and find out what else is going on.

Move Your Body

A gentle exercise will help your circulation moving, flushing toxic fluid. Here's a simple yet effective way that can make a huge difference. Lie on your back close to a wall. Put your legs straight up against the wall and let it stay there for 20 minutes.

Take 2000 mg buffered vitamin C

One to two capsules daily will help relieve the detox symptoms.

Drink Lots of Fluids

Ensure that you are drinking a minimum of 8 glasses every day. You can also drink herbal teas if desired.

Eat!

Eat a lot when you are feeling it. Eat as much of the following non-starchy vegetables:

- Zucchini
- Watercress

- Turnip greens
- Tomatoes
- Swiss chard
- Summer squash
- Spinach
- Snow peas
- Snap beans
- Shallots
- Radishes
- Radicchio
- Parsley
- Palm hearts
- Onions
- Mustard greens
- Mushrooms
- Lettuces

- Kale
- Jalapeño peppers
- Green beans
- Gingerroot
- Garlic
- Fennel
- Endive
- Eggplant
- Dandelion greens
- Collard greens
- Chives
- Celery
- Cauliflower
- Cabbage
- Brussels sprouts
- Broccoli

- Bell peppers (red, green, yellow)
- Beet greens
- Bean sprouts
- Asparagus
- Arugula
- Artichoke

Don't Forget Your Snacks

To keep the hunger and craving away, include 2 snacks in your meal plan. A small protein-based dish with fiber and healthy fats, like sugar-free spreads or dips with veggies or nuts will help keep your energy up and your blood sugar steady. You can also cook your meals, adding a bit of extra to serve as your snack - snack doesn't necessarily mean nuts and spread. If you want, you can eat six small meals a day – some people find this easier.

Set Your Mind

You have to set your mind right. If you are thinking wrong

and if you feel that you won't succeed, then you will head that way. It's not just healthy eating habits; it's also a positive mindset that will determine the success of your detox.

Your journal will help you root out your beliefs, attitudes, and mental obstacles that are preventing you from success. You need to be aware of the challenges so that you can shift your focus to what you want to achieve and how you can reach it.

During your 2-day preparation, focus on the questions below and write whatever comes to your mind. If other feelings and thoughts go to you when you are writing down your answers, then write them down as well. Writing down what happens to your mind makes you more accountable to yourself, and it can transform your inner desires into reality. Here are the questions that you need to answer.

- Why am I detoxifying? What can I achieve in my life and my body with this detox?

- What three particular goals do I want to achieve during this detox?

- What are three particular things stopping me from achieving my weight goal? Is it sugar addiction? Emotional eating? Busy life? Always eating junk food? Fear of failure? Fear of success? Food pushers who advertise and encourage unhealthy food and eating habits?

- What beliefs hinder me from being healthy? Do I think I don't deserve much attention and time? Do I have this belief that being healthy is hard? I tried before, and it wasn't successful.

- Was it the way I overeat? Was it the way I eat food that is not nourishing?

- How do sickness and excess weight affect my ability to fulfill the things I want to do and make me happy?

- If I start eating healthy, how will my life change? If I take care of my health, how will it affect my life?

- How was my life when I was healthier and nurtured myself with care?

The more the obstacles and the benefits come into life, the

better you will be able to get past them. More than that, the more connected you are to your intention and purpose, the more motivated you will be.

Be honest with yourself. Why are you detoxifying? Who are you doing this for? For yourself? For your loved ones? How different will your life be if you are healthy? The most important questions of all – will you be there to witness your children and grandchildren grow up? How long will you be able to spend time with your family and friends?

Measure Your Progress

The day before you start your detox, measure the following and record them in your detox journal.

Weight
Without clothes on, weigh yourself the very first thing in the morning when you wake up.

Height
Measure how tall you are in feet and inches.

Waist Size

Wrapping the tape measure around your belly button, measure the widest point of your waist, not the portion where your belt is located.

Hip Size

Same with the waist, measure the widest point around your hips.

Thigh Circumference

Same with the waist and hips, measure the widest point around each, individual thigh.

Blood Pressure

If you have a blood pressure cuff, then you can do this at home. If not, this can be done at the drugstore or by your doctor.

Now you are ready to start your sugar detox.

Chapter 4: What to Expect and How to Get Through

You are officially starting your sugar detoxification – Day 3 to Day 14. It won't be an easy adjustment and transition. However, if you armed with the knowledge of what to expect and how to tips on how you can deal with the various symptoms, your journey will be more comfortable.

Day 3: This Is It!

This is the when most people usually experience flu-like symptoms, self-doubt, and low blood sugar. This is the start a very challenging journey. Hold on to your reigns! You are likely not experiencing real cold or flu, but you are experiencing the symptoms of sugar detox -this is a typical reaction, and it will subside after a couple of days.

Day 4: Ten More Days to Go!

You may notice your skin breaking out with pimples. This is a normal and a great sign! Your detoxification is working, and your body is clearing out the toxins. You may also experience minor irritation on your skin and mood changes.

Day 5: I made it Through!

The cravings and the headaches will start to go away. If you are unprepared for hunger, slip-ups and temptations may happen. This is what your preparation is all about – having the right food and healthy snacks on hand, plus planning meals on time.

Day 6: Almost Half Way Done!

The flu or cold-like symptoms will begin to subside on this day. You can also check out your supply. The meal plans you have created, and the recipes to make sure you are still on point. It's also good to read the preparation tips once more.

Day 7: One Week Down!

This is where most people experience diarrhea, constipation, or bloating. Make sure you follow the tips given on how to avoid constipation.

Day 8: One More Week!

Over the weekend, you may feel the temptation and slip-off from your detox. If you haven't experienced fatigue early on, then this may be the day you will start to feel worn-out. You might start feeling tired of the food that you are eating and feel overwhelmed by how much preparation you need to do for your food.

If you slipped, don't be harsh on yourself. Instead, be more firm in your commitment. The recipes included in this book are also easy, and there are too many sugar-detox recipes online.

Just make sure each recipe follows the guidelines mentioned above.

Day 9: Yeah! I Am Feeling Good! No More Cravings!

Gas, bloating, and other digestive issues will begin to clear. You may have collected a couple of recipes that you'd like to try and you are getting the hang of cooking. You can change and add any recipes you have clipped outside of this book into your meal plan.

You will also notice that you are no more extended craving more junk and sweet foods the way you did before you started detoxifying. Read your journal. Look back at your successes and your struggles. Your daily log will show you how far you have gone.

Day 10: I Feel A Bit Weak, But This Is Not As Hard As I Thought. I Should Continue Eating Healthy!

A low carb diet can result in weakness or shakiness. If you have been regularly working out, you will notice your performance is affected. Make sure you are getting enough healthy fat. This will be your primary source of energy since you have cut back on carbohydrates and sugar.

After the feeling of lethargy, you will feel the improvement in your energy and mood as you approach the end of your detox. You've now learned to surf on sugar-free waves.

Day 11: I Sleep Like a Baby, But I Am Craving For Something Sweet

By this day, you may notice that you are sleeping faster and better. You will also see that you feel refreshed and rested when you wake up in the morning. Ensure that you follow your waking and sleeping schedule.

However, you may feel the longing for the junk and sugary foods you usually eat, and you may get bored with the food choices. The excitement may pan out at eating healthy food. Again, search for more exciting sugar detox-friendly recipes. You can certainly add tons of recipes to your 2-week meal plan. You can even continue eating healthy for life!

Day 12: Am I Losing Any Weight? The Two Weeks Are Almost Up.

The sugar detox will help you shed the excess weight, but it won't help if you weigh yourself every day. It's ideal to consider yourself once before you start your detox and then after 14 days.

You may feel impatient with only two days to go! Your detox is almost over. Don't think about the detox. Instead, pamper and treat yourself.

See a concert, go to a museum, get a manicure, and see a play. Anything that will distract you from what you are currently doing.

Day 13: Almost Done! What Do I Do After?

You may feel anxious that your detox will soon be over. You will now start planning to reintroduce some of the food that you have eliminated for this detox – beans, and dairy.

You may feel the urge to cheat since your detox is almost over. You may even call it enough since it's already day 13. Keep your goals in mind. This detox is not only about getting rid of sugar, but it's also about changing your unhealthy eating habits into a healthy one. When you make it through just one more day, the feeling of accomplishment will be awesome!

Day 14: I Made It!

Sheer joy! Excitement! Pride! Relief! You pushed through and made it! Tomorrow, you can start reintroducing back the food you were not allowed to eat during the past 2 weeks. Remember to add them back slowly to your diet.

Your Daily Ritual

Here's a reminder of what you need to do every day during your detox.

Morning

- At the start of your day, take your measurements. Write the result in your journal – glucose, blood pressure, etc. Also, take note how many hours of sleep you got and the quality of your sleep.

- Do your 30-minute exercise – brisk walking or your preferred exercise.

- Take your PGX fiber just before breakfast.

- If taking, take your supplement with your

breakfast.

- Optional: Eat your choice of mid-morning snack.

Afternoon

- Take your PGX fiber just before lunch.

- Enjoy your lunch.

- Optional: Eat your choice of a mid-afternoon snack.

Evening

- Take your PGX fiber just before dinner.

- If taking, take your supplement.

- Enjoy your dinner

- Record your experience throughout the day. Jot down what you ate, what you did, how you felt, any changes and improvements in your focus and energy, and how these changes make you feel emotional, mentally, and physically. Write down any detox symptoms.

- Practice your choice of a 5-minute deep-breathing exercise.

- Sleep.

You are now ready to start your detox. Read on through the recipes and carefully plan your meal plan for two weeks. Choose from any of the following recipes or use whatever recipes are sugar detox-friendly.

Chapter 5: Sugar Detox Meal Plan Sample

A sugar detox diet is not as complicated as you think. Just make sure that you stay clear of the foods and products that you need to avoid during the period of your detoxification. Here's a sample of what your meals will look like. It's filled with super delicious real, whole foods that are good for you.

DAY 1	
Breakfast	Spinach and Cheese Baked Eggs
Mid-Morning Snack	Toasted Tamari-Rosemary Almond
Lunch	Sweet Pepper Cheesy Poppers
Mid-Afternoon Snack	3 pieces egg, hard-boiled, remove yolk if desired
Dinner	Baked Spinach-Stuffed Chicken
DAY 2	
Breakfast	Feta and Cucumber Relish

Mid-Morning Snack	Leftover Toasted Tamari-Rosemary Almond
Lunch	Leftover Baked Spinach-Stuffed Chicken
Mid-Afternoon Snack	Cheesy Spinach Dip
Dinner	Asian-Inspired Turkey Lettuce Cups
DAY 3	
Breakfast	Peanut Butter Smoothie
Mid-Morning Snack	3 pieces egg, hard-boiled, remove yolk if desired
Lunch	Leftover Asian-Inspired Turkey Lettuce Cups with Tossed mixed green salad with tomatoes, sweet peppers, cucumber, dressed with vinegar and extra-virgin olive oil
Mid-Afternoon Snack	Leftover Spinach and Cheese Baked Eggs
Dinner	Fresh Herb Marinated Grilled Chicken

DAY 4	
Breakfast	Mini Frittata's
Mid-Morning Snack	1 cheese stick
Lunch	Leftover Fresh Herb Marinated Grilled Chicken with Chicken and Cilantro Salad
Mid-Afternoon Snack	Celery dipped in sugar-free peanut butter or your preferred sugar-free nut butter
Dinner	Bean and Chicken Stew with Mini Cheesy Zucchini Bites
DAY 5	
Breakfast	Leftover Mini Frittata's
Mid-Morning Snack	Mediterranean-Inspired Spicy Feta Dip

Lunch	Leftover Bean and Chicken Stew with Tossed mixed green salad with tomatoes, sweet peppers, cucumber, dressed with vinegar and extra-virgin olive oil
Mid-Afternoon Snack	Tomato, Cucumber, and Feta Salad
Dinner	Cheesy Cauliflower Bread Sticks with Italian-Inspired Green Bean Salad
DAY 6	
Breakfast	Egg Muffin
Mid-Morning Snack	1/4 cup ricotta cheese (low fat, part-skim) tossed with a couple drops liquid vanilla stevia and 1/4 teaspoon vanilla extract
Lunch	Leftover Cheesy Cauliflower Bread Sticks with Italian-Inspired Green Bean Salad
Mid-Afternoon Snack	Mediterranean-Inspired Spicy Feta Dip

Dinner		Lemon-Garlic Chicken Drumsticks with Zucchini Salad
DAY 7		
Breakfast		Scrambled eggs with sautéed mushrooms and spinach with Homemade Salsa
Mid-Morning Snack		1/2 cup cottage cheese
Lunch		Vegetable Soup
Mid-Afternoon Snack		Leftover Toasted Tamari-Rosemary Almond
Dinner		Lemon-Garlic Chicken Drumsticks with Zucchini Salad

Optional After-Dinner Snacks:

- 1/4 cup ricotta cheese (low fat, part-skim) tossed with a couple drops liquid vanilla stevia and 1/4 teaspoon vanilla extract

- 1 cheese stick

- Vanilla-Flavored Chia Pudding

- Cucumber slices topped with cottage cheese (low-fat, about ½ cup)

- 3 pieces egg, hard-boiled, remove yolk if desired

This simple sample meal plan is interchangeable, and you can adapt the recipes to your needs. If you want to customize your meal plan; feel free to search for sugar detox approved recipes and create your special one.

You may be doing this sugar detox solo and will have leftovers. You can scale down the ingredients to adjust the recipe for what you will need for the whole week.

Shopping List

Meats and Eggs	Dairy	Vegetables	Condiments or Miscellaneous
8 ounces pork sausage OR use ground turkey	8 ounces Gouda cheese, OR just use mozzarella	1 bag frozen green beans	1 jar sugar-free natural peanut butter
8 chicken drumsticks	2 packages (8-ounce each) cream cheese	1 bunch of fresh scallions or green onions	1 small-sized jar of sun-dried tomatoes
8 chicken breasts	2 cups Parmesan cheese	1 fresh head cauliflower	2 cans chicken broth, low-sodium
3 dozen eggs	2 cups feta cheese	1 pound fresh green beans	4 ounces chia seeds

1 pound ground turkey	1 package mozzarella cheese, shredded	1 pound mini sweet peppers	Fresh parsley, cilantro, and basil,
	1 package cheddar cheese, shredded	1 stalk celery	homemade hummus for snacking
	1 package cheese sticks	1-2 packages cherry tomatoes	homemade salsa
	1 container (16-ounce) cottage OR low-fat ricotta cheese	18 cups fresh spinach	homemade tomato sauce

		1 container (12-ounce) Greek yogurt, nonfat, plain	4-6 cucumbers	Low-sodium Tamari soy sauce
		1 carton unsweetened almond milk or your milk of choice	6-8 lemons	Powdered or liquid stevia extract
			8 fresh zucchini	Raw almonds
			8 sweet peppers, large-sized	Sesame seeds
			1 package (8 ounces) fresh mushrooms	Vinegar and olive oil to dress salad, also your choice of seasonings

			Frozen spinach	
			Garlic	
			Lettuce leaves for salad and Asian-Inspired Turkey Lettuce Cups	
			Onions, 2 white, and 1 red	

You can follow this meal plan or create your own. You may even know some recipes that are sugar detox-friendly. Feel free to use them.

CHAPTER 6: SUGAR DETOX RECIPES

Spinach and Cheese Baked Eggs

Serves: 6

Prep: 5 minutes

Cook: 15 minutes

Ingredients:

- 6 eggs
- 4 teaspoons olive oil, divided into 2 portions
- 2 teaspoons garlic, minced, divided into 2 portions
- 12 cups fresh spinach, divided into 2 portions
- 1 cup cheese, shredded, divided into 2 portions (I used mozzarella, low-fat)

Directions:

1. Preheat the oven to 350F.
2. Pour 2 teaspoons olive oil into a large-sized skillet.
3. Add 1 teaspoon garlic and 1/2 of the spinach.

Sauté for about 2 to 3 minutes or until wilted. Add 1/2 of the cheese and then stir to combine 2 well.

4. Grease 3 ramekins with nonstick cooking spray. Divide the spinach mixture between the ramekins.

5. Cook the remaining ingredients as directed above and then divide between 3 more greased ramekins.

6. Carefully crack 1 egg over each spinach mixture.

7. Bake in the preheated oven for about 15 minutes for slightly runny yolks or bake until the desired doneness.

8. Season each serving with pepper and salt. Top with some fruit. Serve!

Toasted Tamari Almond Snack

Serves: 4

Prep: 5 minutes

Cook: 5 minutes

Ingredients:

- 2 tablespoons tamari soy sauce
- 1 cup almonds, raw
- 1 tablespoon fresh rosemary, chopped, optional

Directions:

1. Toast the raw almonds in a dry sauté pan over medium heat. Toss and cook until the almonds begin to smell delicious.
2. Remove the pan from the heat.
3. Carefully add 1 tablespoon tamari and, if using, rosemary, into the pan. Return to the burner and cook, continually stirring, until the sauce is absorbed and there are no more juices left.

4. Let slightly chill before serving.

5. Store in an airtight container for up to 7 days.

Sweet Pepper Cheesy Poppers

Serves: 30

Prep: 15

Cook: 15

Ingredients:

- 1 pound mini sweet peppers, halved
- 1/2 cup feta cheese, crumbled
- 1/4 cup onion, grated
- 2 cloves garlic, minced
- 2 tablespoons cilantro, chopped
- 8 ounces cream cheese, at room temperature
- 8 ounces smoked Gouda cheese, grated

Directions:

1. Preheat the oven to 425F.
2. Except for the peppers, put all of the ingredients into a bowl and mix until combined.

3. Fill each sweet pepper half with the cheese mixture.

4. Bake in the preheated oven for 15 to 18 minutes or until the cheese is melty and slight browned.

Baked Stuffed Chicken &Spinach Recipe

Serves: 10

Prep: 10 minutes

Cook: 30 minutes

Ingredients:

- 1 cup frozen spinach, heated, excess water drained
- 1 cup marinara sauce, preferably homemade
- 1 cup ricotta cheese, part-skim
- 1 egg, beaten
- 1/2 cup mozzarella cheese, shredded
- 1/2 teaspoon salt
- 10 pieces (4 ounces) chicken breast, thin, OR 5 pieces (8-ounce) breasts, sliced into halves
- Pepper, to taste

Directions:

1. Preheat the oven to 375F.

2. Put the spinach, ricotta, egg, pepper, and salt into a mixing bowl and combine.

3. Grease a 9x13-inch baking dish with nonstick cooking spray.

4. Put the chicken breast into the greased dish. Evenly divide the spinach mixture between the chicken and put the portions on top of each breast. Roll the chicken and arrange them in the bowl with the seam side facing down.

5. Pour the marinara sauce evenly over the chicken breasts. Sprinkle all over with the mozzarella cheese.

6. Bake in the preheated oven for about 35 to 40 minutes or until the sauce is bubbling and the cheese is melted.

Feta and Cucumber Relish

Serves: 4

Prep: 10 min

Cook: 0 min

Ingredients:

- 1 cup cucumber, peeled and then chopped
- 1 cup fresh tomato, chopped
- 1 scallion, chopped
- 1 tablespoon extra-virgin olive oil
- 1/2 cup feta cheese, crumbled
- Salt and pepper, to taste

Directions:

1. Put all of the ingredients into a bowl and mix until combined.

2. Serve immediately. If not, refrigerate until ready to serve.

Feta and Sun-Dried Tomato Frittata

Serves: 4

Prep: 5 minutes

Cook: 10 minutes

Ingredients:

- 1 clove garlic, minced
- 1/2 cup egg whites
- 1/2 cup light feta cheese, crumbled
- 1/2 cup onion, diced
- 1/2 cup sun-dried tomato, drained, chopped
- 1/4 cup almond milk, unsweetened
- 2 eggs
- 2 scallions, chopped
- 2 teaspoons coconut oil or olive oil

Directions:

1. Put the oil in a medium-sized oven-safe skillet and heat. When the oil is hot, add the onion and garlic. Sauté until the onion is translucent.

2. Add the tomatoes. Cook for about 2 to 3 minutes or until heated through.

3. Meanwhile, crack the eggs, milk, and egg whites into a small-sized bowl and whisk to combine.

4. Pour the egg mixture into the skillet. Evenly sprinkle the feta cheese over the top of the egg mixture.

5. Reduce the heat to low and cook the egg mixture until the middle is almost set and the edges are set.

6. Transfer the skillet to the oven and broil for about 3 to 5 minutes or until the middle is no longer runny.

7. If desired, top with additional feta cheese and scallions.

Spinach Cheesy

Serves: 7   Prep: 5 minutes

Cook: 5 minutes

Ingredients:

- 4 ounces Neufchatel cheese, OR lite cream cheese
- 4 cups spinach, packed into the measuring cup
- 2 teaspoons olive oil
- 1/4 teaspoon salt
- 1/4 cup Parmesan cheese
- 1 cup ricotta cheese, part-skim
- 1 clove garlic, chopped

Directions:

1. Put the oil in a sauté pan and heat. Add the garlic and spinach, Sprinkle with salt and sauté until wilted. Set aside to cool

2. Put the Neufchatel and ricotta cheese into a blender. Blend until the mixture is smooth.

3. Add the Parmesan and cooled spinach. Pulse for 5 to 7 times or until the ingredients are incorporated – DO NOT OVER BLEND.

4. Serve immediately or refrigerate until ready to serve. Serve with your fresh raw veggies kabob– cherry tomatoes, broccoli, peppers, and cucumbers.

Asian Turkey Lettuce Cups

Serves: 4

Prep: 15 minutes

Cook: 20 minutes

Ingredients:

- 1 carrot, large, shredded
- 1 pound ground turkey
- 1 red or yellow bell pepper, large-sized, diced
- 1 tablespoon fresh ginger, minced
- 1/2 cup mushrooms, sliced
- 1/2 cup water
- 1/2 teaspoon salt
- 1/2 teaspoon sesame seeds
- 1/4 cup fresh herbs, chopped: basil, cilantro, or mint
- 1/4 teaspoon Emeril's Asian Essence powder

- 1/4 teaspoon garlic powder

- 1/4 teaspoon ground cinnamon

- 2 tablespoons homemade hoisin sauce

- 2 teaspoons coconut oil or olive oil

- 4 Bibb or Boston lettuce leaves, large-sized

Directions:

1. Put the oil into a large skillet and heat. Add the ginger and the turkey. Cook until the turkey is browned.

2. Add the mushrooms, pepper, hoisin sauce, and water into the skillet. Cook until heated through. Add the Asian essence, cinnamon, garlic powder, and salt. Let heat for 1 minute.

3. Wash the lettuce leaves and dry. Add 1 1/2 cups of the turkey mixture into each lettuce leaf.

4. Sprinkle the turkey mixture with the carrots, herbs, and sesame seeds.

Peanut Butter Smoothie

Serves: 1

Prep: 2 minutes

Cook: 0 minutes

Ingredients:

- 1/2 cup cottage cheese, low fat
- 1/2 cup almond milk, unsweetened
- 1 tablespoon peanut butter, natural, no sugar added
- 1 scoop Whey protein, optional
- 2 full droppers liquid stevia (plain, vanilla, or toffee flavor)
- 1 cup ice

Optional toppings:

- Cacao Nibs
- Peanut butter, to drizzle

Directions:

1. Put all the ingredients in a blender. Blend until the mixture is smooth.

Fresh Herb Marinated Grilled Chicken

Serves: 4   Prep: 10 minutes

Cook: 30 minutes

Ingredients:

- 1 cup mixture of fresh herbs, leaves only, loosely packed (parsley, basil, cilantro)
- 1/4 cup lemon juice
- 1/4 cup olive oil
- 1/4 teaspoon pepper
- 2 large garlic cloves
- 3 pieces (about 1 pound) chicken breasts, boneless, skinless, rinsed, patted dry, sliced lengthwise into halves
- 3 teaspoons salt

Directions:

2. Wash the herbs and then chop them. Put into a high-powered blender or food processor. Add the lemon juice, oil, pepper, salt, and garlic; process until smooth.

3. Put the chicken into a Ziploc bag. Add the marinade, seal the bag, and massage to coat the meat with the marinade. Put the container in the fridge and let marinate for at least 30 minutes and up to 8 hours.

4. When ready to serve, grill the chicken breasts for about 10-15 minutes per side or until cooked through – the meat no longer meat and the juices run clear.

Vegetable Soup

Serves: 8

Prep: 10 minutes

Cook: 40 minutes

Ingredients:

- 1 cup carrots, sliced
- 1 cup green beans, frozen
- 1 cup onion, chopped
- 1/2 teaspoon garlic powder
- 1/2 teaspoon salt
- 1/4 teaspoon pepper
- 2 cloves garlic, large-sized, minced
- 2 cups celery, sliced
- 2 cups fresh spinach, chopped
- 2 cups vegetable stock or chicken broth, low sodium
- 2 teaspoons olive oil
- 4 cups water

Optional:

- 1 cup cannellini beans,
- 1 cup shelled edamame or soybeans
- 1/2 cup fresh parsley, chopped,
- Parmesan cheese, grated

Directions:

1. Put the oil into a Dutch oven and heat over medium heat. Add the garlic and sauté until fragrant.

2. Add the celery, onion, and carrots. Sauté for about 10 minutes or until the veggies are tender.

3. Pour the broth and the water into the Dutch oven and bring to a boil.

4. When boiling, add the green beans and, if using, the soybeans. Add the seasonings.

5. Cover the pot and reduce the heat to low. Simmer for 30 minutes.

6. Remove the cover. Add the parsley and spinach. Cook for about 5 minutes or until the spinach is wilted.

Vanilla-Flavored Chia Pudding

Serves: 2

Prep: 5 minutes

Cook: 0 minutes

Ingredients:

- 1/3 cup chia seeds

- 1 teaspoon vanilla extract

- 1 teaspoon liquid stevia, vanilla flavored

- 1 cup almond milk, unsweetened

- Whipped Cream, dairy-free, optional

Directions:

1. Put all the ingredients in a large pitcher and whisk until combined.

2. Divide between 2 serving glasses.

3. Refrigerate for about 10 minutes or until set.

4. If desired, top each serving with whipped cream.

Notes: You can adjust the amount of liquid stevia. Start with 1/4 teaspoon and increase the amount to taste.

Mini Frittatas

Serves: 12

Prep: 10 minutes

Cook: 30 minutes

Ingredients:

- 8 ounces pork sausage
- 2 egg whites
- 2 cups yellow and red sweet peppers, diced
- 10 eggs
- 1/4 teaspoon pepper
- 1/2 teaspoon salt
- 1/2 cup pepper jack cheese
- 1/2 cup 1% milk

Optional:

- Fresh Cilantro, Chopped
- Green Onions

- Salsa, homemade

- Sour Cream, homemade

Directions:

1. Preheat the oven to 350F.

2. Cook the sausage in a skillet over medium heat until cooked through.

3. With a slotted spoon, transfer the cooked sausage to a plate and set aside.

4. In the same skillet, add the peppers and sauté until soft.

5. Crack the eggs into a large-sized bowl. Add the milk and egg whites. Whisk until combined.

6. Divide the peppers and sausage into 12 muffin cups. Pour the egg mixture into each muffin cup. Sprinkle 1 heaping tablespoon cheese over each.

7. With a fork, stir the contents of the muffin cups to combine.

8. Bake in the preheated oven for about 25 to 30 minutes.

Chicken and Cilantro Salad

Serves: 4

Prep: 10 minutes

Cook:

Ingredients:

- 6 ounces chicken breast, cooked and chopped
- 4 yellow or red peppers, tops cut off and the insides scooped out, OR large-sized tomatoes, cut into halves, and the insides scooped out
- 1/2 cup red onion, diced
- 1/2 cup cherry tomatoes, halved
- 1 cup celery, diced

For the dressing:

- 2 tablespoons fresh cilantro, chopped
- 1/2 teaspoon salt
- 1/2 teaspoon cumin

- 1/2 cup Greek yogurt, nonfat, plain

- 1 teaspoon lemon juice

- 1 teaspoon garlic powder

- 1 tablespoon extra-virgin olive oil

Directions:

1. Put all of the dressing ingredients into a small-sized bowl and mix until combined.

2. Except for the peppers or tomatoes, put the rest of the ingredients into a large sized bowl. Add the dressing and toss to coat.

3. Put about 1 cup of the chicken salad into each tomato half or pepper.

Bean and Chicken Stew

Serves: 12

Prep: 10 minutes

Cook: 3 hours

Ingredients:

- 2 cups chicken, cooked, shredded
- 4 cups chicken broth, low-sodium
- 3 teaspoons garlic, minced
- 1/2 teaspoon salt
- 2 teaspoons cumin
- 1/2 teaspoon oregano
- 1 can hominy or corn, drained and then rinsed
- 1 can black beans, drained and then rinsed
- 1 cup salsa, homemade, OR 1 can diced tomatoes
- 1 can Lima/butter beans, Or cannellini beans, drained and rinsed

- 1/2 cup sour cream, homemade

Optional toppings:

- Fresh cilantro
- Cheese, shredded
- Chives
- Sour cream
-

Directions:

1. Except for the sour cream and the optional toppings, put all of the ingredients into a crockpot. Mix to combine. Cover and cook for 3 hours on HIGH.

2. When the cooking time is up, add the sour cream to the pot and mix until well incorporated.

3. Cover the pot and cook on LOW for 30 minutes.

4. Serve topped with your preferred toppings

Mini Cheesy Zucchini Bites

Serves: 3

Prep: 5 minutes

Cook: 15 minutes

Ingredients:

- 1 egg
- 1/2 cup Parmesan cheese, grated
- 1/4 cup fresh cilantro, chopped, optional
- 2 cups zucchini, grated (about 2 to 3 medium-sized)
- Salt and pepper, to taste

Directions:

1. Preheat the oven to 400F.
2. Grease a mini muffin pan with nonstick cooking spray.
3. Put the zucchini, cheese, egg, and cilantro in a bowl. Mix until combined.

4. Evenly divide the zucchini mixture between the mini muffin cups. Fill each cup to the top, patting them down if needed to pack the cups.

5. Bake for about 15 to 18 minutes or until the edges are golden brown. Check after 15 minutes.

Mediterranean-Inspired Spicy Feta Dip

Serves: 8

Prep: 10 minutes

Cook: 0 minutes

Ingredients:

- 1 cup feta cheese, reduced fat, crumbled
- 1 lemon, juice only
- 1/4 cup almond milk, unsweetened
- 1/4 cup chopped walnuts, toasted
- 1/4 cup Greek yogurt, nonfat, plain
- 1/4 cup red peppers, roasted, chopped
- 1/4 teaspoon pepper
- 1/4 teaspoon Tabasco sauce, homemade
- 2 teaspoons extra-virgin olive oil
- Kalamata or green olives, optional, for topping

Vegetables to dip:

- Celery
- Seedless cucumbers
- Carrots

Directions:

1. Put all of the ingredients into a blender or a food processor. Pulse or blend until the mixture reaches your desired consistency.

2. Transfer to a serving bowl. If desired, top with more olives and red peppers.

3. Serve immediately or keep refrigerated until ready to serve.

Cheesy Cauliflower Bread Sticks

Serves: 4

Prep: 5 minutes

Cook: 40 minutes

Ingredients:

- 1 cup mozzarella cheese, shredded
- 1 cup Parmesan cheese, grated
- 1 teaspoon garlic powder
- 1 teaspoon Italian seasonings
- 1/2 teaspoon salt
- 2 egg whites, OR 1/4 cup egg whites
- 4 cups cauliflower, chopped (about 1 head cauliflower, washed clean and dried)
- Marinara sauce, homemade

Directions:

1. Preheat the oven to 450F.

2. Line 2 pieces of 8x12-inch baking sheets with parchment paper.

3. Microwave the cauliflower for about 7 to 8 minutes or steam for about 20 minutes or until tender.

4. Put the cooked cauliflower into a food processor; pulse until resembling rice.

5. Transfer the cauliflower rice to a large-sized bowl. Add the Parmesan cheese, seasonings, and egg whites. Mix until well combined.

6. Spread the cauliflower mixture into an even layer in one of the prepared baking sheets.

7. Put the baking sheets into the oven and bake for about 30 minutes or until the tops are browned.

8. Invert the cauliflower into the other prepared baking sheet. Put in the oven and Bake for about 10 minutes or until the tops are browned.

9. Sprinkle the top with mozzarella cheese. Broil for about 1 minute or until the cheese is melted.

10. Let rest for 10 minutes and then slice into 24 portions.

Italian-Inspired Green Bean Salad

Serves: 10

Prep: 5 minutes

Cook: 5 minutes

Ingredients:

- 1 1/2 pounds fresh Italian green beans, OR any kind
- 1 cup cherry tomatoes, halved
- 1/2 cup fresh basil, chopped
- 1/2 cup red onion, sliced
- 1/4 cup fresh flat or curly leaf parsley, chopped
- 2 cups English cucumber, sliced with the skin on
- 2 ounces Pecorino Romano cheese, chunks

For the Italian dressing:

- 1 lemon, juice and zest
- 1/2 teaspoon garlic powder

- 1/2 teaspoon salt

- 1/4 teaspoon pepper

- 2 tablespoons extra-virgin olive oil

- 2 tablespoons red-wine vinegar

Directions:

1. Bring a large-sized pot with water to a boil. When the water is boiling, add the beans. Blanch for 5 minutes. Immediately drain and then put the beans into an ice bath – a bowl filled with ice and water. Let fresh for about 5 to 10 minutes.

2. When the beans are chilled, drain and put into a serving bowl. Add the remaining ingredients to the pan.

3. Put all of the Italian dressing ingredients into a small-sized bowl and whisk until combined. Pour the dressing over the salad ingredients.

4. Gently toss to coat. If needed, adjust pepper and salt to taste.

5. Serve immediately or refrigerate until ready to

serve.

Egg Muffin

Serves: 1

Prep: 2 minutes

Cook: 2 minutes

Ingredients:

- 1 tablespoon cheese, shredded, your choice
- 1 tablespoon cream, OR milk
- 1/2 scallion, chopped
- 3 egg whites, OR 1 egg
- Nonstick cooking spray
- Salt and pepper to taste

Directions:

1. Grease a small-sized dish or a custard ramekin with nonstick cooking spray.

2. Put the egg whites/egg and cream into the dish. Whisk to combine.

3. Add the scallion and cheese. Loosely cover the dish with a paper towel and put the plate in the microwave; microwave for about 50 to 60 seconds. If your microwave had a scrambled eggs setting, use that. Do not microwave for too long or you will have a significant mess.

Lemon-Garlic Chicken Drumsticks

Serves: 8

Prep: 5 minutes

Cook: 20 minutes

Ingredients:

- 8 chicken drumsticks
- 3 cloves garlic, minced
- 2 tablespoons olive oil
- 2 lemons, juice only
- 1/4 cup fresh parsley, chopped
- 1/2 tablespoon butter
- 1 teaspoon salt
- 1 teaspoon pepper
- 1 teaspoon dried Italian Seasonings
- 1 lemon, zest only

Directions:

1. Put the olive oil in a large-sized sauté pan and heat.

2. While the pan is heating, season the chicken drumsticks with pepper, salt, and Italian seasoning.

3. When the oil is hot, put the chicken into the pan and cook until all the sides are browned. Transfer the drumsticks to a plate and cover with foil to keep warm.

4. Reduce the heat to low. In the same skillet, add the butter and garlic, stir for about 1 to 2 minutes. Add the lemon zest and juice. Return the drumsticks to the pan.

5. Cover and let simmer for 20 minutes.

6. Coat the drumsticks with the sauce and transfer the drumsticks to a serving plate. Pour the remaining sauce over the chicken. Garnish with chopped fresh parsley. Serve!

Zucchini Salad

Serves: 6

Prep: 10 minutes

Cook: 0 minutes

Ingredients:

- 4 zucchini, medium-sized, shredded (about 6 cups)
- 1 lemon, zest only
- 1/2 teaspoon salt
- 1/4 cup fresh parsley and basil, chopped
- 2 lemons, juice only, OR 3 tablespoons lemon juice
- 3 tablespoons extra-virgin olive oil
- Pepper, to taste

Optional toppings:

- Dried cherries
- Goat cheese
- Almonds, sliced

Directions:

1. Slice, dice, or shred the zucchini to get 6 cups total. Put into a large-sized bowl.

2. Put the oil, lemon zest and juice, pepper, and salt into a small-sized bowl and whisk until combined.

3. Pour the dressing over the zucchini. Add the parsley and basil. Gently toss to coat.

4. If desired, top with extra toppings.

5. Serve immediately or keep refrigerated until serving time.

Homemade Salsa

Serves: 11

Prep: 5 minutes

Cook: 5 minutes

Ingredients:

- 1 can (28 ounces) whole peeled tomatoes, drained
- 1 cup onion, chopped
- 1 cup red pepper, chopped
- 1 tablespoon olive oil
- 1 whole jalapeno pepper, seeds and membrane removed, chopped
- 1 whole lime, juice only
- 1/2 cup fresh cilantro, chopped
- 1/2 teaspoon ground cumin
- 1/2 teaspoon salt

- 2 cans (10 ounces each) diced tomatoes with chilies

- 2 cloves garlic, chopped

Directions:

1. Put all of the ingredients into a food processor. Pulse 5 times for a chunky salsa or vibration up to 10 times for restaurant style.

2. Keep refrigerated.

FINAL WORDS

Thank you again for purchasing this book!

I really hope this book is able to help you.

The next step is for you to join our email newsletter to receive updates on any upcoming new book releases or promotions. You can sign-up for free and as a bonus, you will also receive our "*7 Fitness Mistakes You Don't Know You're Making*" book! This bonus book breaks down many of the most common fitness mistakes and will demystify many of the complexities and science of getting into shape. Having all this fitness knowledge and science organized into an actionable step-by-step book will help you get started in the right direction in your fitness journey! To join our free email newsletter and grab your free book, please visit the link and signup: www.hmwpublishing.com/gift

Finally, if you enjoyed this book, then I would like to ask you for a favor, would you be kind enough to leave a review for this book? It would be greatly appreciated!

Thank you and good luck in your journey!

Alkaline Diet

The Ultimate Beginner's Alkaline Diet Food Guide to Naturally Reclaim & Balance Your Health, Achieve Rapid Weight Loss, Understand pH and Transform Your Body + Fresh, Fast & Delicious Recipes Included!

By *Simone Jacobs*

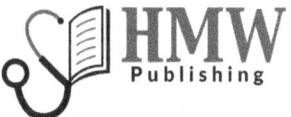

For more great books visit:
HMWPublishing.com

Table of Contents

Introduction..........................9

Dash Notes To The Ash Diet – What Is It Exactly? 11

Chapter 1: Acid-Alkaline Balance 101 - All The Gist You Need To Know About pH and What It Has To Do With Your Health? 13

Health and pH 14

Determining What Affects Your pH 16

Stimulants 17

Exercise 18

Stress 18

Water 20

Personalizing Your Plan 20

Assess Your pH Tendencies (Some People Are Naturally Acidic)............................21

Chapter 2: Acidic Wastes and How High Acid Levels Cause Diseases and Overweight 26

Claim to Bone Loss Due to High Acid Diets 27

Claim to Kidney Stones Due to High Acid Diet 27

Claim to Cancer Due to High Acid Diets 28

When They Say High Acid = High Weight Gain 29

Chapter 3: Symptoms of Having a Low Alkaline Level 32

Heartburn and GERD...................32

Tooth Decay...................36

Blood Sugar Imbalance...................36

Chapter 4: Treatment of Acidosis 39

Chapter 5: Benefits of the Alkaline Diet 41

Preserves Bone Density and Promotes Muscle Mass 43

Lowers Risk of Hypertension and Stroke 45

Helps Enhance Immune Function .. 45

Aids in Lowering Cancer Risk 46

Lowers Chronic Pain and Inflammation 47

Improves Vitamin and Mineral Absorption 48

Maintains Optimal Weight 49

Chapter 6: Good Alkaline Food and Bad Alkaline Food 50

Food to avoid 50

Food to eat to increase alkalinity 51

Bonus Chapter: Delicious Alkalinizing Recipes..................55

- Tomatoes with Quinoa Filling 55

- High Protein Blueberry Spinach Smoothie 58

- Minty Banana Coconut Shake 60

- Lettuce Cups filled with Adzuki Beans and Avocado 62

- Lentil and Thyme Soup 64

- Cucumber Lavender Water ...66

- Watermelon Mint Water 67

- Chilled Watercress With Avocado and Cucumber Soup 68

- Green Curry 70

- Chocolate Mousse with Avocado 72

- Veggie Sticks with Guacamole Dip 73
- Naked Chilli 75
- Kale with Quinoa Salad Served with Lemon Vinaigrette Dressing 78
- Berry Almond Smoothie 80
- Banana Almond Berry Smoothie 82
- Veggie Carrot and Leeks Soup 83
- Veggie Delight Pasta 85
- Brussels Sprouts Salad with Pistachios and Lemon 88
- Pasta Zucchini with Spinach Lemon Pesto 90
- Sweet Potato Soup With a Hint of Curry 92
- Alkaline Power Up Treats 94

- Choco Mint Smoothie 96

- Detoxifying Ginger Lemon Turmeric Tea 98

Conclusion 100

Final Words 102

INTRODUCTION

Recently, massive attention is directed towards Alkaline Diet, as well as a surprising increase in the number of people getting to the bottom of what it is and what makes it so accessible. Most importantly, how efficient it can be to heal your body. In fact, the increased popularity of Alkaline Diet is so impressive that it has resulted in a lot of literature. A quick Google search of "Alkaline Diet" would return 3.18 million results on the topic in a split second. That being said, which writing should you focus your attention? Which ones are worth your time? And which ones would give you the unbiased information you need (without all the hullabaloos and hard to understand science jargons)?

Well, you have made the right decision in picking up this book *"Alkaline Diet: The Ultimate Beginner's Alkaline Diet Food Guide to Naturally Reclaim & Balance Your Health, Achieve Rapid Weight Loss, Understand pH and Transform Your Body + 50 Delicious Recipes."*

This book will walk you through all the essential facts you need to know about the Alkaline Diet. All the necessary things without the hard to comprehend nonsense. Just pure, practical information along with straightforward to follow suggestions on getting into the diet as well as quick fix recipes to get you started with your best foot forward. You will get to learn the importance of a well maintained alkaline digestive system and better appreciate a lifestyle of eating healthily without having to sacrifice a lot. Not only will this book provide you will all the helpful tips to get you started, but will also give you advice as to how to keep maintaining the alkaline diet to ensure your success. The bonus fifty simple recipes will help get you started right away. You don't get a better deal than that!

Also, before you get started, I recommend you joining our email newsletter to receive updates on any upcoming new book releases or promotions. You can sign-up for free, and as a bonus, you will receive a free gift. Our *"Health & Fitness Mistakes You Don't Know You're Making"* book! This book has been written to demystify, expose the top do's and don'ts and to finally equip you with the information you need to get in the best shape of your life. Due to the overwhelming amount of misinformation and lies told by magazines and self-proclaimed "gurus", it's becoming harder and harder to get reliable information to get in shape. As opposed to having to go through dozens of biased, unreliable and untrustworthy sources to get your health & fitness information. Everything you need to help you has been broken down in this book for you to easily follow and to immediately get results to achieve your desired fitness goals in the shortest amount of time.

Once again, to join our free email newsletter and to receive a free copy of this valuable book, please visit the link and signup now: www.hmwpublishing.com/gift

Dash Notes To The Ash Diet – What Is It Exactly?

To put it simply, the Alkaline Diet or the Ash Diet is a form of diet where you consume food that will encourage the formation of alkaline rich products in the body. This diet allows for the slight increase in pH within the system to support and promote a healthier system within the body. As it has been shown that your internal pH is affected by the mineral composition of the food you consume, the rationale of Alkaline Diet is to promote the ingestion of food that will help balance the pH levels of the fluids in our body. Since abnormal pH levels in the body have been linked to disease and illnesses, the idea is by following an alkaline diet we balance our pH and prevent chronic diseases from occurring.

Chapter 1: Acid-Alkaline Balance 101 - All The Gist You Need To Know About pH and What It Has To Do With Your Health?

To better understand how the Alkaline Diet works, it is essential that we first dig into the science that backs it up. I know I have said previously that this book will shy away from all the science gibberish, but I assure you this couldn't be any more simple than your typical high school class. We first need to know how pH balance works. The pH scale which is a numerical measure of a solution's acidity or basicity runs from 1 to 14. Seven would be considered the neutral ground and anything below the seven value is deemed to be acidic while anything above it is alkaline or basic. The human body is highly dependent upon an optimal pH where specific regions or systems has strictly controlled mechanisms to maintain this optimal pH. In fact, much of our bodily functions are so heavily dependent on pH that a slight deviation in the optimal pH range could result in catastrophic results, and in some instances even possibly death. And we're not talking about 2 or 5 point change here, it could be as little a deviation as 0.2-0.5 from the optimal range, and that could mean a life or death situation.

When It comes to human digestion, it is the kidneys that would be in charge of maintaining the pH of the blood very close to a value of 7.4 by either secreting or absorbing specific compounds to regulate the pH. This is the main reason that the system does not support bug down if we suddenly ingested a highly acidic diet, the kidney serves to provide the pH buffering mechanism. However, research has been consistent in showing that a chronic diet of highly acidic food could take its toll in the human body and eventually, over time, this may lead to some health consequences.

Health and pH

What exactly happens to the human body when the pH is

not ideal? First of all, if the pH of the body tends to vary a lot, essential proteins in the body which we call enzymes are affected gravely. Enzymes in the body are responsible for making indispensable reactions to take place, and they can only function in the optimal pH. Whenever they are exposed to either a pH so much higher or so much lower than their optimal pH, the enzymes tend to change its structure and cease to function. This can be disastrous to the body because then we will be inhibiting a lot of required biological functions.

Another importance of a balanced internal pH is protection against microbial pathogens, the bacterial, fungal and viral microorganisms we call germs and continuously invade our bodies. These living organisms to thrive under their optimal pH. Our bodies have been designed to function well under a specific pH, anything below or above that will allow these invasive microorganisms to flourish in our body.

And one other important feature about optimal pH is the condition of the immune system. The immune system consists of an army of white blood cells and other cells designed to engulf and rid our bodies of any threat. These immune system cells are highly dependent on the body's alkalinity or acidity that anything beyond the optimal pH will compromise our immune system and hinder it from performing functionally.

To be able to maintain the slightly central state, the body needs to be in constant work at releasing or absorbing compounds. Most of the reactions naturally occurring within the human body lead to the formation of acidic compounds and the body needs to adjust to that immediately. This condition is further perturbed if we burden our bodies with acid-producing foods in our diet time and time again.

Determining What Affects Your pH

pH is not only determined by the diet that you chose to maintain or even the type of food that you ingest. This condition, like most everything when it comes to a human being's wellness, is also heavily dependent on the holistic lifestyle of the person. Just like everything that is related to health (or more broadly to life), moderation is key. Balance in everything is the solution to keeping a fit physical, emotional and mental physique. Too much of something is just as bad as having too little of one thing. Furthermore, the proper pH would be variable for particular regions throughout your body. A phenomenon that is highly reasonable, given that not all organs would function in much the same way and each intricate process in the human body is involving a lot of sophisticated methods – for this book, we would focus on how pH in our digestive system would affect your wellness. The following factors are some of the most common that would change your digestive system's pH considerably.

Stimulants

The stomach and gastrointestinal tract is a complex system, and to function well in digesting our food intake into smaller molecules that would be more meaningful for nutrient uptake of the body; it needs to be in the proper pH range. Several factors stimulate the secretion of acid in the gastrointestinal tract, and most of these are dependent on things we ingest in our body.

When it comes to acid secretion, high-protein food is more effective stimulants in the body compared to food that is mostly made up of starchy products, carbohydrates or lipids. This means that ingesting high protein nuts, beans, eggs, and meat would better spike up the gastrointestinal tract's acidity than reaching for food that is mostly bread, sugar or fatty food.

Exercise

Exercise has been shown to positively improve the efficacy of digestion and eventually lead to a healthy weight. Different types of training could lead to mixed results and negative impacts on the digestive system. For instance, cardio exercises such as running on a treadmill or riding a bike can help reduce or avoid heartburn occurrences. It has been shown that low impact exercises that promote proper breathing and heart rate can encourage a more healthy bowel movement.

On the other hand, extreme exercises that usually involve high impact and repetitive movements such as heavy bench presses or hanging leg raises or barbell squats could bring more harm than help by causing digestive disorders. Thus it is vital that exercise should also be taken in moderation.

Stress

There is an intricate relationship between the digestive

system and the nervous system where the nervous system could have an elaborate control over the functions of the digestive system, and mostly involving the secretion of hydrochloric acid in the stomach. This is the reason why your stomach would be triggered to secrete acid in preparation for a meal as soon as you see, imagine or smell food. This kind of stimulation is not dependent on the food but is mostly dependent on the nervous system's perception. In this same way, stress, where high levels of stress hormones are released in the body, could also profoundly affect the acidity of the stomach and eventually every part of the digestive system. Stress can cause the shut down of the digestive system because the central nervous system shuts down as well. This decreases secretion in the digestive system and eventually the inflammation of the gastrointestinal system, making the body all the more susceptible to infection.

To aid in digestion, we must always keep our stress levels in check and under control. Relaxation therapies are available for dealing with stress issues, and quite possibly the best means to deal with stress is to limit altogether or avoid the cause of stress.

Water

The common conception is that water would dilute digestive juices. This is a reasonable notion, given that water is the universal solvent. Water aids in the proper digestion of food, but by itself, it cannot prompt absorption. However, the intake of ionized or alkalinized water is a different aspect. It has been said that ionized water has had established effects that promote proper digestion but only not within 20 minutes of a meal, this includes before and after ingestion. This is because it has been shown that the high levels of ions in the alkaline water could interfere with the acidity of the digestive system and this, in turn, would cause problems with food digestion.

On the one hand, drinking alkaline water before or after the 20-minute time frame is thought to be good practice for a more healthy digestive tract.

Personalizing Your Plan

With all the advantages of keeping a healthy pH, it is

highly necessary that we know how to keep up with our acidity or alkalinity. The trick is knowing that not everybody type is the same so each of our bodies would react to a particular trigger differently. In the following section, we will be learning about how easy it is to measure our body's pH and then we will learn some practical tips about how to assess our pH tendencies.

Assess Your pH Tendencies (Some People Are Naturally Acidic)

It is highly essential that we test our body's pH because it will not only give us a sense of where our body is in the pH zone. It will also get a clue whether it is gearing towards metabolic acidity, or balance, or is more alkaline than what is to be expected as optimal for our body type.

The best, and possibly most straightforward and most practical, a method for determining your body's pH is to test for your body's excreted fluids like saliva or urine. All you need to have to decide this is a way to measure it. Now, there is the more sophisticated way of measuring pH where you use laboratory grade equipment called a pH meter that would have this probe that you need to dip into your solution of interest for you to be able to quantify the pH as accurately as possible. Fortunately for us, we don't have to go through all the complexity and suddenly feel like we're going into our high school science lab again. Luckily, we can use a tool as simple as paper.

pH papers are available pieces of documents that have been designed specifically for the detection of pH. It would have all these indicators that would change a different color depending on the acidity or basicity of your liquid. All you have to do is wet this pH paper with your solution, wait a couple of seconds and compare the color change in the strip of pH paper with the indicated pH value.

In testing our body's present pH state, it is best that you perform this test in the morning before you have taken your breakfast to record your body's steady state pH without the influence of food yet. So, do this test the first thing in your morning routine after you wake up – and as much as possible, when you have had a good restful sleep of at least 6 hours, this is to make sure that stress is not affecting your pH readings.

To do this test using urine samples, you could collect your

morning's first urine in a cup and dip the strip of pH paper to determine your body's pH. Another option is to do the test using your saliva. Among the two samples, research has shown that the former is better, especially if the urine sample is the first one released after at least six hours of sleep. Saliva is less adequate just because there are a lot more enzymes in the saliva sample and also because urine samples would be coming directly from inside of the body.

To test your pH using saliva samples – again, note that this is best done using samples taken first thing in the morning – take a mouthful of water and gargle and rinse your mouth with it. Spit out the wash and then collect some of your salivae using a spoon. Dip the pH paper strip into the sample of saliva and wait for the color to change and stabilize. It is essential that you do not brush your teeth, eat or drink anything yet before you perform the test, remember we are trying to establish your body's present pH.

Do these simple tests to monitor your body's pH. Although you do not need to measure your pH daily, it would be nice to incorporate this simple morning routine into one of your weekends. Do this test once or twice a week and keep a record of your pH changes. It is especially important if you have the goal in mind to control your body's pH – which I assume would be your case since you are now holding this book in your hand.

Also, an important note is that while others, more often than the other, may start out with an acidic pH with values lower than 6.5, this is entirely normal. Especially given the kind of diet an average American would have nowadays. All you have to do is increase your pH by increasing your intake of fruits and vegetables, nuts, root crops, spices and seeds and all in the effort of improving your alkalinity. Lucky for you, this book will help you achieve that with a lot of practical tips and easy to make recipes.

On the other hand, if your pH is above the 7.5 mark, suggesting highly alkaline steady-state pH then this could be due to high levels of nitrogen in your urine or saliva sample. This is observed when there is more than the usual catabolism or the natural breakdown of specific body tissues. The benefit of having to measure your body's pH routinely is for you to at least keep track of your body's changes. If your readings have been consistently close to the 8.0 pH mark, then you should contact your health professional and seek advice as to how to manage tissue repair and avoid the too much catabolic state in your body.

Chapter 2: Acidic Wastes and How High Acid Levels Cause Diseases and Overweight

Nutrition plays a lead role in the overall wealth of a person, and taking in the wrong kinds of food could lead to deterioration of the human body. We need to be very careful with how we take care of our bodies because despite it's millions of years of evolutionary advantage and learning to cope with any attack there is, our bodies are still very much susceptible to harm. And the most efficient and most silent attacker to our health is the food we intake. We might not be aware, but the little by little amounts of greasy fries, or slimy burger patties or burning alcohol may be enough to accumulate and eat up through our systems.

When it comes to highly acidic diets and its link to some diseases, here are just a few of the most significant impacts acidic diets do to our bodies:

Claim to Bone Loss Due to High Acid Diets

When you have too much acid within your system, you tend to develop chronic acidosis, and this disease has been linked in many studies to bone diseases due to decrease in bone density. Too much of the acid, highly abundant in proton molecules in the body, in the blood, would mean that your body would tend to compensate for this pH drop by attempting to increase it. And the way the body responds to it is by releasing calcium ions from the bones into the blood. Calcium ions are rare alkaline minerals. Having chronic acidosis, however, would tend to deplete the bones from the much-needed calcium they need to establish bone density and this, in turn, results in bone loss and diseases.

Claim to Kidney Stones Due to High Acid Diet

It has been shown that people who are suffering from a chronic kidney disease could have a higher risk of their disease progressing into and eventually developing into kidney failure when they routinely have highly acidic diets. High acid diets are rich in meats and have been linked to this progression to kidney failures. In fact, chronic kidney disease patients have three times higher risk of developing kidney failure as compared to their high alkaline consuming counterparts. People should pay more attention to this tendency, especially if they are already at a risk of kidney diseases.

Claim to Cancer Due to High Acid Diets

There have been a sufficient amount of data out there that would provide the link between pH and cancer. In papers published, they would present researchers that support how cancer would thrive in an acidic environment. This is as a result of cancer cells releasing too much lactic acid, in contrast, it is in the acidic environment that cancer cells would start to have a more significant chance of reproducing. Studies say that as the body begins to accumulate acid-forming substances, the body starts to release materials that would try to circumvent the drop in pH. Over time these elements become toxic to the cell as oxygen levels drop, and the hereditary DNA and respiratory enzymes start getting affected. The natural tendency of the battery is to enter into the physical cell death or apoptosis since the cells are no longer beneficial to the body, they are more of a liability than an asset. However, some cells survive, and instead of entering into normal cell suicide would become abnormal cells having the ability to withstand high levels of acid substances in its environment. The abnormal cells become what we know as malignant cells that are no longer responding to the nervous system, nor to the body's control of gene expression of its DNA. So instead, these cancerous cells start reproducing and making more and more copies of itself, growing indefinitely and without and control until it has become cancer. That silent killer that is devastating millions of the world's population now.

When They Say High Acid = High Weight Gain

There is an intricate relationship between the body's fat and the body's acidity. Although this fact seems to escape a lot of people, putting all the blame into the well marked "culprit" fat, it may be, so that body acidity has much to do with a person's body weight, or maybe even be the mastermind culprit after all. So how do we make sense of this? Wait a minute, isn't obesity measured by the excess amount of fat you have after all? So it is right to blame it all on the fat!

Well, not entirely true. The thing is when your body is experiencing too much acidity; it starts to produce all these toxins that are profoundly harmful to the body. As we've seen above it can lead to bone loss diseases, kidney failures or cancer. It has even been linked to premature aging, diabetes and a lot of other problems. In response to this possible threat, the body tries to protect itself by creating fat cells that would serve as storage vessels for these toxins, absorbing the excess acidic substances and preventing it from further causing harm to the body. It follows that the more acidic materials the body produces, the more fat cells will be needed to store these toxins.

So, in a nutshell, the best way to look at this is if you do not have a lot of junk that you have to store then there would not have to be a lot of these large compartments. To begin with, If you did not have a lot of the harmful acidic substances that act as toxins, then your body would not need to produce more fats. So maybe the next time you start pinpointing at your fats for giving you a horrible time trying to fit into your jeans from last year, maybe start looking at the real cause of the problem and kickstart at rethinking your diet.

Chapter 3: Symptoms of Having a Low Alkaline Level

Heartburn and GERD

Heartburn is one of the most common medical problems that Americans are experiencing on a monthly basis, up to 40% of Americans report to suffer from this condition regularly. It has become part of an average American's lifestyle that one would easily shrug off the problem as soon as it persists thinking that it is merely one of those days where you had something "bad" to eat. As soon as that burning and scorching acidic sensation broils inside your chest, the first go-to treatment of any ordinary American would be a quick discomfort relief – the most popular being the handy Pepto-Bismol. But heartburns should not be shrugged off quickly, the underlying reason for having these heartburns may be more severe than you think and more so if the problem persists more frequently than usual.

The burning sensation one feels as a result of heartburn is caused by the reflux of acid-laden contents in the stomach as a consequence of having a faulty esophageal valve that keeps contents of the stomach from coming back up. Heartburn is the primary and noticeable side effect of low alkaline diet, and this can lead to a number other more life-threatening problems to a person.

The more severe form of heartburn is called Gastroesophageal Reflux Disease or GERD; this occurs when an individual is experiencing chronic heartburns, and uncontrolled persistence of this disease can lead to significant health issues that could damage your teeth and esophagus.

The esophagus links your mouth to your stomach, and when acid from the stomach flows back up, this sets the stage for swelling and irritation of the esophageal lining. The inflammation can make it very hard for a person to swallow and is a health condition called esophagitis.

On the one hand, when GERD continues to persist it will eventually cause sores in the epidermal walls of the esophagus, this makes GERD the leading cause of ulcers.

Associated symptoms of esophageal ulcers could include chest pain, nausea along with the pain accompanied by swallowing.

When inflammation obstinately continues, over time the swelling can lead to permanent damage and eventual scarring of the esophageal lining. Building up of this scar tissue in the esophagus would narrow the esophageal tube and create constricted regions called the esophageal strictures. These make it even harder to swallow food and liquids which eventually leads to weight loss and dehydration. This is a severe problem and should not be taken lightly. Treatments include a procedure that helps loosen the strictures by gently stretching the esophagus.

One other serious problem associated with acid reflux is called Barrett's esophagus, and about 1 out of 10 people with GERD develop this condition. This issue is caused by stomach acid making precancerous changes in the epidermal (outer or surface lining) cells of the esophagus. This increases the risk for esophageal cancer, luckily only 1 out of a hundred people with Barrett's esophagus was found to have esophageal cancer. Still, this should not be taken for granted since the condition does not lead to any apparent symptoms and chest pains which are usually associated with esophageal cancer typically appear only in later stages of the disease when it has progressed. It is nevertheless best to seek professional advice if you have had more than the usual bouts of acid refluxes and heartburns recently. To be able to rule out cancer for certain, endoscopy may be needed wherein a thin, flexible tube with a camera at the tip and linked to the computer enables a health professional to view the insides of your esophagus.

Tooth Decay

This symptom is mostly related to the above condition of having acid flow back into your mouth from the stomach. Heartburns as a result of low alkaline diet can also take a levy on your dashing smile. Stomach acid, like most acid, is highly corrosive and can wear down the teeth's hard outer covering that serves as a protective layer called enamel. The enamel gives us our pearly white smiles and helps us prevent plaque buildup and cavities, without it the teeth weakens and turns yellow.

Blood Sugar Imbalance

Some symptoms associated with sugar imbalance as a result of low pH levels include stubborn headaches that would only go away after eating. Also, there are bouts of energy swings during the day where you may start out with such a high energy and switch to being too tired and over fatigued in a matter of hours without even exerting too much effort. Low pH levels could also increase cravings for simple sugars, carbohydrates and loads of sweets as this provides immediate relief to sugar discomfort. There are also those episodes of blocking out or zoning out after a meal or what millennials like to call "food coma." Coffee addicts may have to beware of their dependence on coffee may also be due to low alkalinity. And lightheadedness could also result in an effect of missing meals.

The imbalance of sugar in the body is a result of your body not being able to handle its fuel source – glucose – efficiently. For proper function, the body needs to metabolize, digest and break down glucose and maintain blood glucose levels at an optimal range. Anything below this may cause lightheadedness as this provides less glucose to the brain especially.

On the one hand, having too much glucose would lead to what we call "sugar rush" where a person experiences episodes of high energy vents. The fluctuation is getting too high energy swings during or after a meal to very low energy swings when you skip a meal, and your body runs out of its food reserve.

Chapter 4: Treatment of Acidosis

To accurately correct the real cause of the problem, the doctor needs to be able to determine the patient's condition and only then can he or she be able to provide with the right kind of treatment for acidosis. There are however some temporary immediate relief treatments that can be used for any types of acidosis regardless of what causes it. One of the most popular treatment is the oral ingestion of sodium bicarbonate (baking soda or generically known pharmaceutically as an antacid). This will help increase the blood pH temporarily and is a preferred go to drug as it can be purchased over the counter and can be taken in orally or some forms can be done via an intravenous (IV) drip.

Acidosis that are affecting the respiratory tract can be treated by targeting the airways and provide relief to the lungs. Drugs designed to dilate the airways can be prescribed, or devices that enable a patient that has obstructed breathing or weakened respiratory muscles to breathe better can also be given to a patient. Devices such as these are called CPAP (Continuous Positive Airway Pressure) devices.

Acidosis that have been associated with kidney failure could also be treated explicitly with sodium citrate to help ease problems with kidney stones. Improper blood sugar balance that results from pH imbalance could be treated with IV fluids and insulin to maintain pH levels to the optimum; this is especially necessary for patients already suffering from diabetes mellitus or ketoacidosis.

Chapter 5: Benefits of the Alkaline Diet

Many types of research would continue to support the many benefits of taking in alkaline inducing diets. In fact, research has shown that from our early ancestors, a lot has considerably changed with our diet coming from a hunter-gathering system to our present condition where the majority of our food intake now would consist of fast food choices and high sodium and high-fat content. Average food intake from hundreds of years past used to be high in potassium, magnesium, and chloride. Until the uprising of the agricultural revolution where humans need not move around to hunt for their food anymore, and instead, they have learned to grow and care for their food. And then followed by the mass industrialization where food businesses would start to improve and people would rely on other businesses to serve their food instead. This shift up to today has increased the sodium intake of people.

Typically it would be the task of our kidneys to help

maintain this electrolyte imbalance or shift – electrolytes such as the magnesium, calcium, potassium, and sodium. When the body is dealing with high acidity, the body will use these electrolytes to fight against bitterness.

Whereas potassium used to outnumber sodium in an average human's diet, this has now dramatically shifter to almost threefold. Increasing in sodium would mean that we have less of the required electrolytes, antioxidants, essential vitamins and fiber to ward off or level out the acidity. To top it all off, the typical diet of the western world is concentrated with refined fats, sodium, simple sugars and chloride.

All of these changes have inevitably led to an increase in metabolic acidosis, a condition where the pH levels of the human body are no longer optimal. Many are now suffering from a deficient nutrient intake, with micronutrient deficiencies for potassium and magnesium.

Metabolic acidosis increases the aging process and would eventually lead to gradual loss of organ functions and degeneration of bone mass and many tissues.

On the one hand, there is still hope because the effects of

highly acidic substances in the body could be very simply reversed by changing our diets and rethinking about how we treat food consumption.

If the risks of having highly acidic internal body system will not persuade you enough to enter into an alkaline diet, then this following list of the benefits of alkaline diets would hopefully, finally, do the trick.

Preserves Bone Density and Promotes Muscle Mass

The development and maintenance of bone structure are highly dependent on the intake of minerals. A myriad of researchers has linked the consumption of more alkalizing vegetables and fruits to a better response of the body in protecting against decreased bone strength and muscle wasting as the body continues to age. This wasting of the body's muscle and bones is a condition called sarcopenia.

An alkaline diet helps to balance the ratios of minerals necessary and crucial for bone building and lean muscle mass maintenance. These minerals include not only the well-known calcium but magnesium and phosphate as well.

Alkaline diet not only helps in mineral balance, but it also helps improve the production of growth hormones and vitamin D absorption. These biomolecules are essential players that help protect bone loss and also contribute heavily to lessening many other chronic diseases.

Lowers Risk of Hypertension and Stroke

One of the well-known effects of engaging in an alkaline diet is the response to anti-aging, and the diet does this by decreasing inflammation in the body, consequently increasing the production of growth hormones. Increase in growth hormone and reduction in inflammation has been shown to improve cardiovascular health by preventing a lot of the commonly reported problems such as hypertension caused by high blood pressure, high cholesterol content, stroke, kidney stones and even memory loss.

Helps Enhance Immune Function

The body's first defense to get rid of harmful elements in the body is to properly dispose of them as wastes, expel them out of the body or convert them into less toxic substances. However, when the body, particularly the cells, lack enough of the crucial minerals that would help them perform this function, the entire body would suffer. The absorption of vitamins is hugely compromised by the loss of essential minerals. As a result, toxins and pathogens (germs such as bacteria, virus or fungi) start to accumulate in the body and as a result systematically weaken the immune system.

Aids in Lowering Cancer Risk

A lot of peer-reviewed research publications have shown that cancerous cell death, or the condition we technically call apoptosis, was more likely to occur in a body that is high in

alkalinity. This proves that this links cancer prevention to a high alkaline diet. Indeed, the process of preventing cancer development is now believed to be connected with a shift in pH towards a more alkaline end due to an alteration in the electric charges and the release of basic components of proteins. Not only is an alkaline diet beneficial for people who have not yet developed cancer by lowering their risk for it. An alkaline diet has also been shown to provide people being treated for cancer or recovering from its treatments, with a better chance of ridding themselves of it. An alkaline diet has been shown to be more beneficial for a lot of chemotherapeutic chemicals and drugs that usually need a higher pH for it to work more efficiently.

Lowers Chronic Pain and Inflammation

Still much more other studies have revealed the link between a high pH diet with that of reduced levels of chronic pain. On the one hand, constant acidosis has been found to contribute to a lot of chronic pain disorders such as muscle spasms, chronic back pain, menstrual cramps, headaches, joint pains, and inflammation.

One significant study that has been performed by experts in Germany has shown that supplementing alkalinity to some patients suffering from chronic back pain in four weeks have shown a substantial decrease in pain for seventy-six out of eighty-two patients involved in the study. Although the mechanism for this preventive action has not yet been fully elucidated, apparently the link is there for a better lifestyle with the alkaline diet.

Improves Vitamin and Mineral Absorption

Magnesium is an essential systematic cofactor for thousands of enzymes required to perform some metabolic processes. The increase in magnesium content is therefore beneficial for a lot of bodily processes. Many people are, unfortunately, suffering from magnesium deficiency and mostly due to the choice in diet. The consequences of this lack are heart complications, headaches, muscle pains, anxiety and sleep disorders. Magnesium is one of the crucial elements required for vitamin D activation, necessary for the overall immune and endocrine function of the body.

Magnesium is present in a bulk of highly alkalinizing food, and thus just by increasing this food intake, you are already doing your body a tremendous amount of favor.

Maintains Optimal Weight

Limiting the intake of highly acid forming foods and instead shifting to higher consumption of more alkaline forming food can protect you from developing obesity. This is by decreasing the number of leptin levels in the body as well as inflammation. Leptin affects a person's cravings and is usually the culprit being blamed for why we reach for a second serving almost instantly after a meal. Inflammation and leptin levels also affect the body's fat burning abilities. Daily intake of the anti-inflammatory alkaline inducing foods would allow your body to reach normal leptin levels and help you fell satisfied and full easily and longer. Preventing you from overeating and only reaching for the right amount of calories you really need.

Chapter 6: Good Alkaline Food and Bad Alkaline Food

Food to avoid

Here are some of the food you need to eat less of if you find out that your pH is lower than the normal range. These food increase acidity and should be taken sparingly.

- Carbonated or soft drinks (soda)
- Dairy products such as cheese (especially parmesan and sharper cheese), milk and yogurt
- Simple Sugars
- Simple carbohydrates such as white bread, rice, and pasta
- Meat (Pork, chicken, beef, lamb) and fish – these should be taken in moderation
- Grains such as oats, cornmeal, wheat, rye, bran

and spelt

- Grain products such as cereals, pastries, crackers

- Unsprouted beans (sprouted beans are alkaline forming foods): mung, navy, lentils, garbanzo, white, red, adzuki, broad

- Sunflower and pumpkin seeds

- Nuts such as pecans, walnuts, cashews, macadamias, pistachios, peanuts and brazil nuts

- Alcoholic beverages

- Caffeinated drinks

- Sweeteners (artificial or natural like barley syrup, honey, maple syrup, molasses, fructose)

- Soy sauce and table salt

- Mustard, ketchup, and mayonnaise

- White vinegar

Food to eat to increase alkalinity

These alkalinizing food list will help you neutralize the

effects of eating foods that lower pH.

Here are some of the most common ones:

- Vegetables (practically all of this product are alkalinizing)

- Fruits (interestingly citrus fruits (rich in ascorbic acid or vitamin C and citric acid) are alkalinizing, only avoid cranberries, blueberries, prunes, and plums)

- Beans (especially sprouted ones) such as soy, green, lima, string and snap

- Peas

- Potatoes

- Exotic grains such as quinoa, millet, flax, and amaranth

- Nuts such as almonds and chestnuts

- Sprouted seeds of radish, chia, and alfalfa

- Unsalted butter

- Eggs

- Whey
- Herbal teas
- Garlic
- Cayenne pepper
- Gelatin
- Miso
- Vanilla spices
- Brewer's yeast
- Cold-processed and unprocessed oils

It is important to note that just because they are acid-forming, they should not be avoided altogether, in fact, many of these acid-forming food are necessary for healthy metabolism and proper body function. The key to utilizing this list of different pH regulating food is to know when to eat one kind sparingly and know when to eat more of the other. Again the most important thing when it comes to diet and health is the balance. The following chapter will help you appreciate the alkaline diet better with some fun and simple recipes that help give you the best out of your food selections.

Bonus Chapter: Delicious Alkalinizing Recipes

- Tomatoes with Quinoa Filling

SERVINGS: 4

INGREDIENTS

4 large tomatoes

2 cups quinoa seeds

6 cups baby spinach

4 cloves of garlic, minced

1 can kidney beans (rinse and drain)

¼ cup basil, (cut into thin strips)

2 tbsp. coconut oil

4 cups water

sea salt

black pepper to taste

PREPARATION

Turn on oven and set to 375 degrees, allow to reach temperature. Empty the insides of the tomatoes by making about a quarter inch slice on the top of the tomato and scooping out the inside contents with a spoon. Make a small cut off the bottom of the tomato to allow it to sit flat on a baking pan (Make sure not to cut too thick and ruin you're hollowed out tomatoes). Drizzle a little salt into the insides of the tomatoes.

Combine 4 cups of water with the quinoa seeds and cook the quinoa in a pot set on top of the stove on high heat. Allow the water to come to a boil and turn the heat down to the minimum setting and cover the pot. Keep cooking the quinoa seeds for an additional 30-45 minutes.

In another pan set on top of the medium heat, drizzle the coconut oil and fry garlic until it is lightly browned. Pour in the kidney beans into the pan and using a spatula, slightly crush them on the pan. Allow the beans to cook for about 1 -2 minutes. Pour in the baby spinach and as soon as they cook and wilt, add the basil. Season with salt and pepper.

In a large bowl, pour in your spinach mixture and cooked quinoa seeds. Carefully stuff your spinach-quinoa filling into your hollowed-out tomatoes. Line a baking pan with wax paper and place your stuffed tomatoes on top. To prevent your tomatoes from drying up too much, sprinkle a little water (about 5 tbsp). Bake tomatoes for about 25 minutes. Plate, serve and enjoy!

High Protein Blueberry Spinach Smoothie

SERVINGS: 2

INGREDIENTS

1 cup blueberries

2 cups baby spinach

2 Tbsp. almond butter

2 Tbsp. chia seeds

2 Tbsp. ground flaxseed

2 Tbsp. hemp seed powder

2 Tbsp. coconut oil

4 cups almond milk

PREPARATION

Blend in blueberries and spinach in almond milk, add the chia seeds, ground flaxseed, and hemp seed powder. Blend until seeds are consistent with the mixture. Add almond butter and coconut oil and blend on high to make the smoothie. Serve and enjoy! (Optional: this could be served with a little sprinkle of mint on top)

Minty Banana Coconut Shake

SERVINGS: 2

INGREDIENTS

2 cups coconut milk

1 cup spinach

½ cup fresh mint leaves

2 bananas, frozen

4 dates, pitted

1 tsp. vanilla

sea salt to taste

Optional: ¼ tsp. Mint extract, and/or ¼ tsp. peppermint extract

PREPARATION

Blend spinach, mint leaves, and banana into coconut milk. Make sure to thoroughly blend the spinach and mint leaves. Add in the frozen bananas and dates and blend on high. Add a teaspoon of vanilla and a small dash of sea salt to taste, mix and add more if desired. You may add in the mint and/ or peppermint extract before pouring into tall glasses. Serve and enjoy! (Optional: This fancy drink is best served with a little drizzle of chocolate flakes and coconut cream on top)

- Lettuce Cups filled with Adzuki Beans and Avocado

SERVINGS: 2

INGREDIENTS

15-ounce can of Adzuki beans (drain and rinse)

1 avocado

1 head romaine lettuce

¼ cup minced red onion

¼ cup chopped cilantro leaves

1 lime

Sea salt to taste

Red pepper flakes (optional)

PREPARATION

In a bowl, pour in Adzuki beans and red onions and mash them together until consistent. Pour in the chopped cilantro leaves and stir until thoroughly mixed. Season with salt. Cut out romaine lettuce and form into cups. Add a spoonful of the bean and onion mash into the lettuce cups. Dice the avocado and garnish on top of the bean and onion mash. Finish with a squeeze of lime juice. Plate, serve and enjoy! (Optional: To add a little zing to every bite, sprinkle red pepper flakes before serving)

- Lentil and Thyme Soup

SERVINGS: 4

INGREDIENTS

1 tbsp. extra virgin olive oil

1 medium onion, finely chopped

4 garlic cloves, minced

2 large carrots, chopped

2 stalks of celery, chopped

6 cups of vegetable broth

1½ cups brown lentils, rinsed

1 bay leaf

1 tsp. thyme

Small handful of parsley, chopped

Sea Salt and pepper to taste

PREPARATION

Heat a drizzle of oil in a large pot on a stove set to medium heat. Add chopped onion and fry until it turns a little brown. This will take about 5 minutes. Add carrots, garlic, and celery and fry for another 3 to 5 minutes. Mix the lentils, thyme, bay leaf into the vegetable broth and pour in the mix into the large pot. Cook soup on medium to low heat or until the lentils are tender enough. This will take about 40 minutes. Salt and pepper to taste. Stir in parsley. Serve and enjoy hot!

- Cucumber Lavender Water

SERVINGS: 4

INGREDIENTS

1 tbsp dried lavender

8 pints water

1 medium-sized cucumber

PREPARATION

Cut cucumber into thin slices. Combine lavender, sliced cucumber and water in a pitcher and refrigerate for about half a day, or enough to let the lavender and cucumber blend in the mix. Serve and enjoy! (This is perfect for that distressing moment)

- Watermelon Mint Water

SERVINGS: 4

INGREDIENTS

8 pints water

1 medium-sized watermelon

¼ cup mint

PREPARATION

Cut watermelon into cubed slices. Combine mint, cubed watermelon and water in a pitcher and refrigerate for about half a day, or enough to let the mint and watermelon blend in the mix. Serve and enjoy!

Chilled Watercress With Avocado and Cucumber Soup

SERVINGS: 2

INGREDIENTS

6 organic avocados

4 scallions

1 medium-sized cucumber

4 cups of watercress

2 lemons, freshly squeezed

3 cups of filtered water

Salt and pepper to taste

1 cup Cherry tomatoes

PREPARATION

Dice cucumber and half cherry tomatoes. Blend the cucumber, watercress, avocados, and scallions with half the water. Once the mix has turned into a thick puree pour in the rest of the water. Add lemon squeezes, salt, and pepper to taste. Continue to blend until consistent. Pour into bowls, garnish with cherry tomatoes, serve and enjoy!

Green Curry

SERVINGS: 4

INGREDIENTS

¼ cup coconut oil

1 large onion, peeled and diced

3 tbsp. green curry paste

1 cup green beans

1 large broccoli crown, cut into florets

1 cup snow peas

1 medium-sized Brussels sprouts, halved

4 cups garbanzo beans, cooked or canned

2 15oz. cans of unsweetened coconut milk

4 pints vegetable broth

1 bunch kale

1 bunch bok choy

Salt and pepper to taste

Fresh cilantro for garnish

PREPARATION

Drizzle large pot with coconut oil and sauté onions with curry paste until the onions are brown and tender. This will take about 10 minutes. Add green beans, broccoli, peas, Brussels sprouts, garbanzo beans and coconut milk. Combine and allow to simmer. Wait about 15 minutes. Add the vegetable broth and continue to simmer until all the vegetables have turn tender. Another 15-30 minutes. Add the kale and bok choy and season with salt and pepper. Take out of the heat. Plate with cilantro, serve and enjoy!

- Chocolate Mousse with Avocado

SERVINGS: 2

INGREDIENTS

1½ Haas avocado

2/3 cup freshly squeezed coconut water

1 tbsp. vanilla

2 tbsp. raw cacao

3-5 dates

1½ tsp. Sea Salt

PREPARATION

Blend avocado with the coconut water until consistent. Add vanilla, cacao, and dates. Continue to blend on high. Add salt and mix. Pour, serve and enjoy!

Veggie Sticks with Guacamole Dip

SERVINGS: 4

INGREDIENTS:

2 avocados

2 tbsp plum tomato, finely chopped

2 tsp white onion, chopped

2 tsp freshly squeezed lime juice

2 tsp. jalapeño, diced

2 tbsp cilantro, finely chopped

2 cloves of garlic, minced

½ tsp sea salt

PREPARATION

In a bowl, mix the cilantro, onion, and jalapeño and add the salt. Using either a pestle or a large spoon, mash the ingredients together.

Add avocados to the mashed ingredients and using the pestle or a fork, mash in the avocados to the mixture. You don't have to thoroughly mash the avocados; it should just be smooth enough to blend with the ingredients but still have a little chunky texture. Stir in the finely chopped tomatoes, lime juice, and salt to taste. Serve with the mix of your veggie sticks on the side. Enjoy!

- **Naked Chilli**

SERVINGS: 4

INGREDIENTS:

2 cups tomatoes, chopped

½ tsp. thyme

2 cups soaked sun-dried tomato

½ tsp thyme

½ tsp sage

1 cup cherry tomatoes

1 tsp cumin

1 tsp paprika powder

1 tsp chipotle powder

1 tsp chili powder

1 tomato, diced

¼ cup cilantro, chopped

¼ cup carrots, diced

½ cup red onion, diced

¼ cup celery, diced

¼ cup zucchini, diced

½ avocado, diced

2 garlic cloves, minced

2 scallions, diced

1 tsp jalapeño, diced

5 basil leaves, chopped

salt to taste

PREPARATION

Place all the different kinds of tomatoes into a food processor (with the "S" blade if possible) and cut for a few consecutive times. Switch the food processor to blend and add all the vegetables, as well as the garlic, jalapeño, cilantro and other powdered spices. Blend the mixture until consistent enough to liking.

Pour into a bowl and let the mixture sit for an hour. Serve with the avocado and scallions as garnish and enjoy!

Kale with Quinoa Salad Served with Lemon Vinaigrette Dressing

SERVINGS: 4

INGREDIENTS:

½ cup sliced almonds

½ cup pomegranate arils seeds

½ cup cooked (boiled) quinoa seeds

4 cups chopped kale

3 tbsp freshly squeezed lemon juice

¼ cup olive oil

1/4 cup apple cider vinegar

zest of lemon

PREPARATION

To prepare the dressing, whisk together the apple cider vinegar, olive oil, lemon juice and lemon zest in a small bowl and set aside.

Prepare the salad by placing the kale in a large bowl and top with quinoa, avocado, almonds and pomegranate seeds. Toss the salad (or if you want you can pour the dressing on top before tossing it, or serve with dressing on the side). Combine salad well. Salt and pepper to season. Serve and enjoy!

- **Berry Almond Smoothie**

SERVINGS: 2

INGREDIENTS:

½ cup frozen strawberries

1 cup frozen blackberries

1 ½ cup almond milk

2 tbsp coconut oil

1 lime, freshly juiced

1 large bunch of kale

½ tsp vanilla

1 tbsp raw almond butter

PREPARATION

Blend in kale into the almond milk, allow to reach desired consistency. Mix in the blackberries and strawberries, coconut oil, lime, kale, vanilla and almond butter.

Continue to blend until you make a smoothie. Serve in tall glasses and enjoy!

Banana Almond Berry Smoothie

SERVINGS: 2

INGREDIENTS:

1 frozen banana

4 tbsp raw almond butter

1 cup frozen mixed berries or strawberries

2 cups almond milk

2 cups fresh spinach

PREPARATION

Start by blending the spinach with the almond milk until you reach desired consistency. Add the banana and mixed berries or strawberries. Continue blending and add the raw almond butter. Pour smoothie into a tall glass, serve and enjoy!

- **Veggie Carrot and Leeks Soup**

SERVINGS: 4

INGREDIENTS:

2 carrots

3 weeks with the green parts removed

1 thinly sliced fennel bulb

1 cup thinly sliced savoy cabbage

4 cloves minced garlic

3 tbsp coconut oil

a handful of chopped parsley

1 can kidney beans, drained and rinsed

6 cups vegetable stock

2 fresh rosemary sprigs, leaves removed and chopped

sea salt and pepper

PREPARATION

Heat a large soup pot over stove over medium-low heat. Add oil and leeks, fennel and carrots and allow vegetables to cook or until leeks are soft enough and slightly browned. This will usually take about 7 minutes.

Add the rosemary and garlic and allow to cook for another minute or so. Next, add the cabbage and sauté for another minute or two.

Pour in the vegetable stock into the mixture and allow to boil. As soon as the stock boils, add the beans and cook on low heat for about 15 minutes or until all the vegetables have gone tender.

Stir in the parsley into the soup and season with salt and pepper to taste. Pour into individual bowls, serve and enjoy!

Veggie Delight Pasta

SERVINGS: 4

INGREDIENTS:

1 package of kelp noodles

1 can kidney beans, drained and rinsed

1 medium head of broccoli

1 thinly sliced leek

1 spring of chopped rosemary

1 handful chopped parsley

½ tsp red pepper flakes

3 cloves minced garlic

3 tbsp extra virgin olive oil (or coconut oil)

salt and pepper

PREPARATION

Preheat oven to 400 degrees and allow to reach temperature. Toss the broccoli in garlic, red pepper flakes, extra virgin olive or coconut oil and salt. Roast the entire mix into the oven for 20 minutes or until the vegetables are tender enough upon touch with a fork.

While the vegetables are roasting, rinse and drain kelp noodles and soak in a pot filled with hot water. Meanwhile, heat 2 tablespoons of the extra virgin olive or coconut oil in a frying pan and add the leeks. Cook leeks in the pan until it has melted. This will usually take about 10 minutes.

Drain the kelp noodles and continue cooking by adding them to the melted leeks. Cook together for another 10 minutes.

Combine roasted broccoli mix into the pan. Add the parsley and rosemary. Add salt and pepper to taste in the mix.

Mix in the kidney beans. Plate in a salad bowl, serve and enjoy!

- Brussels Sprouts Salad with Pistachios and Lemon

SERVINGS: 4

INGREDIENTS:

16 large Brussels sprouts (end of the sprout cut off and leaves peeled off from the core)

¾ cup shelled pistachios

zest and juice collected from one lemon

2 tbsp. extra virgin olive oil

salt and pepper to taste

PREPARATION

Drizzle oil on a large skillet or wok and place on top of the stove to heat on medium-high for a few minutes. Add the pistachios to the skillet (or wok) and the lemon zest. Sauté mix for an entire minute before you add the Brussels Sprouts leaves. Toss the mix until Brussels sprouts are bright green enough but still crisp. This will take about 5 minutes.

Squeeze lemon juice over the mixture. Toss and season with salt and pepper. Plate in a salad bowl, serve and enjoy!

Pasta Zucchini with Spinach Lemon Pesto

SERVINGS: 2

INGREDIENTS:

4 zucchinis

3 cups baby spinach

Juice of 1 small to medium lemon

½ cup cherry tomatoes, sliced in half

½ cup extra-virgin olive oil

¼ cup cashews

3 garlic cloves

¼ cup basil

PREPARATION

Using a spiralizer, make zucchini pasta by making it into long strands. This is best done using raw zucchini or flash sautéed for two minutes.

Meanwhile, in a food processor with an "S" blade, mix in spinach, garlic, basil and cashews, and pulse until finely chopped. Keep the food processor on and slowly add in the lemon juice and olive oil.

Season with salt and pepper to taste.

Toss the freshly prepared zucchini pasta and spinach lemon pesto together. Garnish the dish with cherry tomatoes. Plate in a large salad bowl, serve and enjoy!

- Sweet Potato Soup With a Hint of Curry

SERVINGS: 4

INGREDIENTS:

3 peeled sweet potatoes, cut into 1-inch cubes

2 tsp. curry

2 cups water

1 15oz can of full-fat coconut milk

zest and juice of one lime

4 cloves garlic, minced

1 ½ inch piece of ginger, sliced and crushed

1 tbs. coconut oil

½ bunch cilantro, chopped

PREPARATION

In a large saucepan, add coconut oil and heat pan on the stove over medium heat. Add the garlic, ginger and lime zest and cook until the garlic is slightly browned. This will take about 5 minutes.

Add curry to the pan and cook until fragrant. Normally takes another minute.

Stir in coconut milk and water along with sweet potatoes. Bring mixture to a boil and reduce to low and simmer. Cover for about 25 more minutes and allow to simmer.

Turn the heat off and leave the pot on the stove for about a half hour to allow flavors to blend.

Using a blender or a food processor, puree the soup. Garnish the final puree with chopped cilantro and dash with lime juice.

Serve in a bowl and enjoy!

- Alkaline Power Up Treats

SERVINGS: 3

INGREDIENTS:

1 cup hulled hemp seeds

2 tsp vanilla

3 tsp cinnamon

¼ cup cacao nibs

3 tsp chia seeds

¼ cup flax seeds

6 pitted dates

1 cup raw almond butter

PREPARATION

Mix in the a processor the cup of raw almond butter and six pitted dates.

Add the rest of the remaining ingredients into the food processor except for the hemp seeds. Continue pulsing until you have created a ball in the food processor.

Using your hands, roll mix into inch-sized balls and then coat the treats in hemp seeds as well as the 3 teaspoons of chia seeds.

Store the balls in an airtight container. These treats are good for up to a week. Plate on a plate, serve and enjoy!

Choco Mint Smoothie

SERVINGS: 2

INGREDIENTS:

1 cup of frozen coconut water

1 tsp chia seeds

½ small avocado

½ cup packed mint leaves

2 tbsp cacao nibs

1 cup almond milk

4 pitted dates

¼ cup raw almonds

PREPARATION

Start by blending the coconut water ice with the cup of almond milk and avocado scoops. Add the rest of the mint leaves, cacao nibs and dates. Pulse until you have created a smoothie. Pour into tall glass, garnish with chia seeds, serve and enjoy!

Detoxifying Ginger Lemon Turmeric Tea

SERVINGS: 2

INGREDIENTS:

1 lemon slice

pinch of black pepper

1 inch of fresh organic ginger root

1 inch of fresh organic turmeric root

about 20 oz water

PREPARATION

Bring water in a pot to a boil. While the water is boiling, peel the turmeric and ginger and dice them into small pieces. The size would depend on your preference for taste, the smaller the dices, the more flavourful the tea would be.

Once the water has boiled, remove the pot of water from the heat and add turmeric, ginger and black pepper to the pot. Replace pot on the stove and simmer for another 10 minutes. This again would depend on how strong you would want the tea. The more you simmer, the stronger the flavor.

Pour into a cup and serve with a squeeze of lemon. Leftovers can be stored in an airtight container in the fridge and can be served as iced tea. Enjoy!

Conclusion

Whether it is to improve your weight or reduce your risk of developing all the diseases and disorders that are associated with metabolic acidosis, or that condition where your body's pH is below the optimal range. Your decision to ditch the high fat, simple sugar diet and switch to the high alkalinity inducing one is probably the best favor you have done your body just yet.

As you have seen throughout the book, and as we have continued to emphasize and justify in the book, backed up with a lot of scientific research and real-life practical claims. The alkaline diet is definitely for you! It does not matter whether you are a fully pledged stay at home mom, or a hardworking young male professional with the stead nine to five routine. Or a recovering cancer survivor or a senior citizen with some struggles with chronic muscle pains, then the alkaline diet can be your solution to achieving the body and health you have been striving for. It does not even matter how young you are, because as it shows you are never too young to enter into the alkaline diet. There are no restrictions or limitations.

I hope that this book has helped encourage you to dive into the alkaline diet and sooner experience all the benefits associated with this beautiful not so secret.

And as a parting gesture, we salute and congratulate you on your journey towards self-growth, improved health and better lifestyle.

FINAL WORDS

Thank you again for purchasing this book!

I really hope this book is able to help you.

The next step is for you to join our email newsletter to receive updates on any upcoming new book releases or promotions. You can sign-up for free and as a bonus, you will also receive our "*7 Fitness Mistakes You Don't Know You're Making*" book! This bonus book breaks down many of the most common fitness mistakes and will demystify many of the complexities and science of getting into shape. Having all this fitness knowledge and science organized into an actionable step-by-step book will help you get started in the right direction in your fitness journey! To join our free email newsletter and grab your free book, please visit the link and signup: www.hmwpublishing.com/gift

Finally, if you enjoyed this book, then I would like to ask you for a favor, would you be kind enough to leave a review for this book? It would be greatly appreciated!

Thank you and good luck in your journey!

Intermittent Fasting

The Ultimate Beginner's Guide To The Intermittent Fasting Diet Lifestyle - Delay, Don't Deny Food - Finally Lose Weight, Burn Fat, Live A Healthier & More Productive Life

By Simone Jacobs

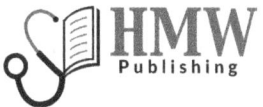

For more great books visit:
HMWPublishing.com

Table Of Contents

Chapter 1: Lose Weight and Build Muscle on a Time-Tested, Ancient Healing Tradition 12

    Gear Your Body, Mind, and Spirit towards Healing and Weight Loss 13

    A Brief Glance at the History of Fasting 14

    Modern-Day Fasting 15

    Fasting is not Starving 16

    Teach Your Body to Burn Glucose and Fat 18

    Recalibrating a System Dependent on Food 18

    Make Your Body into a Sugar-and-Fat-Burning Machine 20

    Fasting is the Easiest Way to be Healthy 24

Chapter 2: The Virtues of Intermittent Fasting 28

Decrease Insulin Levels 30

Boost Weight Loss 31

Burn Belly Fat Faster 33

Stimulate the Production of Growth Hormone 33

Increase Adrenaline Levels 35

Regulates Functions of Cells, Hormones, and Genes 37

Repair Cells 37

Alters Gene Expression 38

Relieve Inflammation 38

Develop Strong Heart 39

Anti-Aging 40

Improve Your Focus and Mental Clarity 41

Release Energy for Healing 43

Fosters Spiritual Growth 45

Reasons Why Fasting Works 46

Relaxing 46

Lengthens Life Span 47

Complement Chemo Therapy 48

Chapter 3: Effectively Adapting to the Healthy Change 50

Electrolyte Deficiency 50

Uric Acid Elevation 52

After-Fast Weight Gain 54

Lean Muscle Mass Loss 56

Not Everyone Can Fast 57

Those Who Shouldn't Fast 57

Fasting for Women 59

Intermittent Fasting Options for Women 60

Crescendo Method 61

Chapter 4: Listen to the Needs of Your Body 67

Buffer Your Weight Loss and Muscle Gain Journey 67

Start Your Diet with a 1-Day Fruit or Juice Fast 68

#1 - Leangains Method (16:8 Fasting) 70

#2 - Eat Stop Eat (24-Hour Fasting) 72

#3 - The Warrior Diet (20/4 Diet) .. 74

#4 – Fat Loss Forever 76

#5 - UpDayDownDay (Alternate-Day Fasting) 77

#6 – Fast Diet (5:2 Fasting) 79

#7 – Daniel Fast 80

Chapter 5: Successfully Transitioning into a Healthier You 83

Prepare for the Detoxification and Ketosis Symptoms 83

Disrupted Sleep Patterns and Fatigue 84

Headache 84

Nausea 85

Cravings and Hunger 86

Stay Hydrated 86

Prefer Overnight Fasting 86

Transform Your Thinking Process ..87

Start When You're Busy 87

Hit the Gym 87

Conclusion 90

Final Words 92

About the Co-Author 94

Introduction

Do you have a weight loss problem? Do you continuously watch out for answers in the market hoping for a quick and efficient solution to your problem? If you do, then this book is entirely right for you!

Everyone seems to be in a rush searching for ways to weight loss nowadays. A myriad of offers covering dieting, health and food supplements, physical fitness programs, and various training workshops are flooding the entire health and fitness market. All these entail costs and effort on your part and mostly turn out to be not as effective as these marketers promised in their glamorous ads.

However, there's an ongoing solution that many are resorting to nowadays. Although it is not exempted from cynic opinions, it is a lot better than those options being offered in the market. For one, it does not require your extra effort to do it, and it does not hit your pocket like it does when you prepare for a new set of diet or enrol in a physical fitness program.

The popularity of intermittent fasting is gaining momentum in the market today when people are getting tired of numerous diets that sound easy to do at the first attempt but usually do not work well in the long run.

This book, "*Intermittent Fasting: 7 Beginner's Intermittent Fasting Methods for Women & Men-Weight loss and Build Lean Muscle Hacks*" is designed to provide you with an efficient alternative solution to your problem regarding weight.

This book will further enlighten you about the fundamentals of Intermittent Fasting and how it proves to be the coolest, quickest, and easiest way to lose weight while building lean muscles for both men and women. Grab a copy of this book before it's gone and start dropping pounds in fewer days!

Also, before you get started, I recommend you joining our email newsletter to receive updates on any upcoming new book releases or promotions. You can sign-up for free, and as a bonus, you will receive a free gift. Our "*Health & Fitness Mistakes You Don't Know You're Making*" book! This book has been written to demystify, expose the top do's and don'ts and to finally equip you with the information you need to get in the best shape of your life. Due to the overwhelming amount of mis-information and lies told by magazines and self-proclaimed "gurus", it's becoming harder and harder to get reliable information to get in shape. As opposed to having to go through dozens of biased, unreliable and un-trustworthy sources to get your health & fitness information. Everything you need to help you has been broken down in this book for you to easily follow and to immediately get results to achieve your desired fitness goals in the shortest amount of time.

Once again, to join our free email newsletter and to receive a free copy of this valuable book, please visit the link and signup now: www.hmwpublishing.com/gift

Chapter 1: Lose Weight and Build Muscle on a Time-Tested, Ancient Healing Tradition

The demands and responsibilities of life often lead to various health problems, especially when you are too distracted and you overlook the importance and the practice of a healthy lifestyle and eating habit. More often than not, you do notice the slow changes happening to your body, but you are too busy to do anything about it. The only time you will ever really decide to do something about your concern is when you are already getting sick to the point that you cannot work efficiently.

So your search for solutions begins, but which diet, training, and health fitness program REALLY works? There are tons and tons of them out there. The answer is simple. Teach your body to heal itself and to lose weight by learning when to eat and when to stop eating.

Gear Your Body, Mind, and Spirit towards Healing and Weight Loss

Learning when to eat and when to stop eating is a practice called Intermittent Fasting (IF). This concept is nothing new. It's a method used by many people all over the world since time immemorial. Humans go through long periods without eating for most of our history for various religious reasons and when the food source is scarce. In fact, when we sleep, we inadvertently fast.

We fast when we sleep? Yes, indeed! If you typically eat your dinner by 8 pm and have your breakfast at 8 am the morning you wake up, you are fasting for 12 hours and eating for 12 hours. We call this fasting method as a 12/12 fast. Isn't that great news? You can fast while sleeping! I mean it's no effort at all if you choose to practice this method.

But fasting is not exclusive to humans, even animals fast when they are ill or stressed, and sometimes when they feel slightly uneasy. Fasting is a natural tendency for every organism, whether animal or human, to conserve energy during critical times and to seek balance and to rest.

A Brief Glance at the History of Fasting

Hippocrates, Galen, Socrates, Plato, and Aristotle, as well as early great healers, thinkers, and other philosophers all praised the benefits of fasting for healing and health therapy. Paracelsus, one of the three fathers of Western medicine said, "Fasting is the greatest remedy--the physician within."

Early spiritual and religious groups fast as part of their rites and ceremonies, especially during the fall and spring equinoxes. Almost every dominant religion observe fasting for various spiritual benefits.

North and South American Indian traditions, Hinduism, Buddhism, Islam, Gnosticism, Judaism, and Christianity use one form of fasting or another for sacrifice or mourning, penance, spiritual vision, or purification.

Yogic practices, including fasting, date as far back as back as thousands of years. Paramahansa Yogananda, a famous yogi and guru said, "Fasting is a natural method of healing." Likewise, Ayurveda, ancient healing practice, includes fasting as part of its therapy.

However, scientific medicine became dominant and developed better drugs. Fasting and other Naturopathic ways of healing fell off the stage. Recently, many people searching for health solutions return to the old ways.

Modern-Day Fasting

The time-tested, ancient healing tradition of intermittent fasting is back in the spotlight and gaining popularity among many people today. Between 1895-1985, Herbert Shelton, a physician, followed and supervised the fasts of over 40,000 people. During the century and concluded that fasting is a radical and fundamental process that is older than any practice of healing the body, an instinctive method when an organism is sick.

Even though IF is a practice that is as old as the human race itself, modern science and recent studies now reveal that knowing when and eat and when to stop eating creates significant positive changes in the body, resetting the entire system that increases its ability to function at high levels both mentally and physically. Indeed, many research supports the health benefits of IF.

Food abstinence keeps the mind and memory sharp, reduces the risk of various diseases, and keeps the body cells healthy. A study titled, "The Scientific Evidence Surrounding Intermittent Fasting" conducted by Amber Simmons, Ph.D., pointed out that IF together with caloric restriction, is an effective method to promote weight loss in obese and overweight individuals.

Fasting is not Starving

When people hear the word fasting, they often think of it as synonymous to starving. This misconception can often lead people astray and choose other never-been-heard, exotic, and sometimes complicated, diet method.

Starving is when you don't know when your next meal will come. On the other hand, fasting is a practice where you strategically plan periods of when to 'eat' and 'stop eating.' In fact, the word breakfast is the meal you eat to break the fast that you do every day while you are sleeping.

Moreover, it is not the fasting but the caloric restriction that comes with limiting what you eat that produces the health benefits. For example, if you eat at 6 am in the morning and refrain from eating anything within the next 9 hours, then you are actually restricting your calorie without counting, given that you only eat the right amount of food and do not eat double servings of your meal at breakfast. The key to IF is 'discipline,' not starvation.

Teach Your Body to Burn Glucose and Fat

Intermittent Fasting is not a diet per se, but a method in which you teach your body to compartmentalize into "eating" and "fasting" periods. How does learning when to eat and when not to eat help a person lose weight?

Recalibrating a System Dependent on Food

The body metabolizes fat and glucose from the food you eat as its primary source of energy. Carbohydrates are the primary source of glucose. When you eat carb-rich diet, they are broken down into the simpler form called glucose. This substance circulates freely in the bloodstream into every cell of your body as the energy source. When you eat, you supply your body with enough glucose to sustain your body with enough energy to run for 3-4 hours.

Excess glucose goes to the liver and muscles for storage and becomes the body's secondary source of energy. When the cells run out of free circulating blood glucose, the body will break down and metabolize the stored glycogen and transforms it into glucose. Glycogen is the reason you do not have to eat every 15 to 20 minutes. In fact, glycogen stores in your body can sustain you for 6 up to 24 hours after your last meal.

The problem begins when you consume excessive amounts of carbohydrates. Your body runs out of storage capacity for glycogen, so the liver converts it into adipose tissue, triglycerides, or fat for long-term storage. And because you continuously supply the body with energy by eating 3 meals and 2 to 3 snacks in between, the cells consistently have an excess supply of glucose, which is converted into more glycogen in the liver and fat in the body.

Do you see the picture clearer now? Most of us consume more energy than our body can utilize, so the system stores them as glycogen and body fat. We also tend to eat when we feel slightly hungry, so we do not give our cells the chance to use these stored fuels. Thus, we end up adding more and more stored glycogen and adipose tissue into our system, which leads to various health problems, including diabetes, overweight, and other related illnesses linked to high-sugar and high-fat content in the body.

Moreover, when we eat continuously, your body is used to the constant supply of free-circulating glucose, which could lead to insulin resistance. It is a condition where the body is repeatedly with high levels of sugar and insulin in the blood until your system no longer produces sufficient insulin to metabolize glucose or become resistant to its effect.

Make Your Body into a Sugar-and-Fat-Burning Machine

The simple principle behind intermittent fasting is "discipline." **Not feeding or eating for periods gives the body a chance to burn off excess and stored glucose and fat. Practicing IF recalibrates your body from a system that**

is dependent on food into a sugar-and-fat-burning machine.

The human body is a fantastic mechanism with a developed system that allows it to deal with periods of low food source. It undergoes the 5 sequent process or stages below to sustain the need for energy.

Feeding

Eating food raises the insulin levels of the body, allowing the tissues of the body to utilize the glucose as energy. During this stage, the liver stores it any excess as glycogen within itself. When the storage space of glycogen in the liver is full, the organ transforms the surplus it into triglyceride or fat for extended storage.

Glycogen Breakdown

Within 6 to 24 hours after your meal, the insulin level will start to fall. During this period, the body will begin metabolizing the stored glycogen as energy and this secondary source of glucose in the liver can sustain the body for about 24 hours.

Gluconeogenesis

After roughly 24 hours up to 2 days without a ready source of glucose, the body utilizes amino acids, the simple form of protein, to manufacture new glucose during the process called "gluconeogenesis." In a non-diabetic person, the glucose levels will fall but stay within the normal range.

Ketosis

After 2 to 3 days without food, the low insulin levels in the body stimulates the breakdown of triglycerides or stored fat for energy during the process called lipolysis. The body metabolizes the stored fat into 3-fatty acid chains and glycerol backbone. The body uses the glycerol for gluconeogenesis or manufacturing of new glucose. The body tissues can readily utilize the 3-fatty acid chains as energy.

However, the brain cannot, so the body metabolizes the 3-fatty acid chains into ketone bodies or energy that can pass in the blood-brain barrier as the brain's fuel source, which is mainly in the forms of acetoacetate and beta-hydroxybutyrate, to sustain the brain's energy needs.

Four days after the body's last meal, 75 percent of the energy used by your mind is from ketones, and the amount increases over 70 times during the fasting period.

Protein conservation

On the 5th day, fasting stimulates the production of growth hormone to help the body maintain lean tissue and muscle mass. During this period, the metabolic system utilizes ketones and fatty acids entirely as the source of energy. The level of adrenaline (norepinephrine) also increases to adapt to the change, giving the body more fuel.

Of course, you will not be depriving yourself of food nor be starving during intermittent fasting. As mentioned, IF practice focuses on scheduling when to eat and when not to feed, which gradually teaches the body to utilize excess and stored sugar and fat as energy instead of relying on food. This traditional method opens the gates to better health, weight loss, and building of muscle mass and lean tissue.

Fasting is the Easiest Way to be Healthy

The best thing about intermittent fasting is you can incorporate it into any healthy and balanced diet. When diet is particularly hard to follow, you have the option to stop worrying about what to eat at the very least. It is also convenient when you do not have to prepare meals for a period. Plus, you can save on some amount of money, too. But that's not the real reason why most people love intermittent fasting. There is more to the practicality IF practice offers.

Some people developed the habit of not eating healthy food choices and unhealthy feeding patterns throughout their lifetime, including eating in between meals, choosing fast and junk foods over a well-balanced diet, or just routinely giving in to constant food cravings when they feel hungry. All these constitute an unhealthy lifestyle, which can eventually lead to serious health problems.

Going on a diet and doing a fasting practice both leads to weight loss; hence, people aiming to shed their excess fat face a predicament when choosing which method to adapt to a healthier lifestyle.

According to Dr. Michael Eades, co-author of the famous book, "Protein Power," it is always easy to contemplate on a diet, but it is often harder to execute. Contrary to an eating program, intermittent fasting is just the opposite, it appears to be too hard to contemplate, but once you perform, you find it is not that hard at all.

Going on a diet is always easier during the first few days, but the longer you stay on it, you find it less and less appealing. The reason why most diets do not work out in the long run. Only a few people manage to integrate one form of eating into their lifestyle.

Thinking of fasting would always send you to believe you can't survive a day without eating, especially for those who badly need to fast. However, you will find it easier to do when you start doing it. Turning it into a habit and making it a part of your lifestyle is easier done than just contemplating on it. It's hard to overcome the idea of not eating, but once you go over the hurdle, intermittent fasting is, in fact, easier to do than following a diet.

Intermittent fasting acts as a reset button. It does not regulate nor does not tell you what kind of food you should eat and not consume. Instead, it determines the best time when you should have a proper, healthy, and well-balanced meal. It's an eating pattern that you integrate into your lifestyle to recalibrate your body and improve your health.

Key Takeaways:

- Fasting is a time-tested, ancient healing tradition that can help you lose weight and build muscles.

- The practice of scheduling your feeding time gears your body, mind, and spirit towards various health benefits.

- The key of intermittent fasting is discipline, not starving. It is simply planning when to eat and when not to eat.

- Fasting with caloric restriction recalibrates your body from a sugar-fueled system into a fat-burning machine.

- It resets the button, giving your body the chance to relax and direct energy for healing, weight loss, and muscle building.

Chapter 2: The Virtues of Intermittent Fasting

Before you start fasting, you need to understand what hormonal adaptation your body will undergo concerning fat loss, so you do not immediately plunge into it just to stop before it even starts working on your body.

For starters, let's review the "fed state" and the "fasted state" of the human body. A human body is in a fed state when it is taking in and digesting food. Generally, the feeding starts at the time you start eating the food, and this will last for 3-5 hours while your digestive system is working on it.

While in the fed state, your body cannot burn fat efficiently because of the high level of insulin in the body that enables the sugar to be utilized by the cells as energy.

However, after the digestion process, your body will soon be in the post-absorptive state, which means that your body is no longer working on processing a meal. This period will last from 8 to 12 hours after your last meal, and during this period, your body starts to gain entry to the fasted state. It is during this time that your body begins to burn fat, and your insulin level will begin to lower.

Take note that your body only enters the fasted state 12 hours after your last meal, and since most of us eat 3-6 meals a day, it is rare that your body is getting into this condition; hence, you are depriving your body of experiencing the fat-burning state.

The reason why those who are practicing IF were able to lose fat even without changing the kind and the quantity of food they are eating or how often they have their exercise. Intermittent fasting allows your body to undergo the fat-burning process that you rarely experience when you have your regular eating schedule.

Intermittent fasting maximizes the glycogen and fat-burning mechanism of the body. During the "fasting state," your system undergoes various hormonal adaptations that lead to weight loss and muscle gain.

Decrease Insulin Levels

All food raises the insulin levels in the body. Therefore, the most consistent, efficient, and effective strategy for lowering it is to avoid foods. If you are a non-diabetic person, your blood glucose levels remain normal as your body starts to switch into fat burning. This adaptation is evident in as short as 24-36 hours of fasting. The longer you fast, the longer the duration of reduced insulin and the decrease is more significant.

According to a study titled, "Alternate-day fasting in nonobese subjects: effects on body weight, body composition, and energy metabolism," fasting every other day is an effective method to reduce insulin levels without affecting the normal glucose levels of the body.

Fasting decreases insulin level by 20-31 percent and lowers your blood sugar by 3-6% once your body utilizes stored fat starts as fuel in place of carbohydrates, thus, likewise reducing the risk for Type 2 diabetes.

Boost Weight Loss

Another reason why intermittent fasting is popular these days is that scientific studies prove it is a powerful technique for weight loss. We love to eat food rich in carbohydrates and fats, and then we panic once we see our weight measurement rise.

With an IF practice, you can choose between eating fewer meals or entirely not consume any food for a few days. This process is sure to reduce the overall calorie intake, as well as normalize the hormonal change that inhibits fat burning as it triggers the release of norepinephrine (noradrenaline).

Through short-term fasting, you can increase your metabolic rate up to 14 percent. Intermittent fasting likewise results in weight loss by changing your caloric equation, e.g., taking in fewer calories and burning more of it.

The same study that showed the effects of alternate-day fasting in reducing insulin levels further revealed after 22 days, the 16 people who ate every other day lost 2.5 percent of their body weight.

The study further showed that their hunger increased during the first fasting day and remained high. There was no significant change in their resting metabolic rate (RMR) and respiratory quotient (RQ) from day 1 to day 21, but on the 22nd day, their RQ decreased, which resulted in a significant increase in fat oxidation or loss in their bodies up to 15 grams and more.

However, since hunger on fasting days did not decrease, the authors of the research suggested that eating a small meal during fasting days make this approach more acceptable. Nevertheless, the study corroborated that fasting is an efficient and fast strategy to lose excess weight.

Burn Belly Fat Faster

Belly fat or what we call the "love handles" are the most dangerous of all the fats stored in your body. The name may sound appealing, but love handles are very sinister. They are hazardous visceral fats that tend to build around the internal organs and later lead to severe illnesses.

However, a study revealed that undergoing intermittent fasting not only reduce body weight; it also decreases waist circumference by 4 to 7 percent.

Stimulate the Production of Growth Hormone

Growth hormone (HG) or somatotropin or human growth hormone (HGH or hGH) stimulates cell reproduction and regeneration and growth, thus, is very vital to human development. It is a natural hormone produced by the pituitary gland, and the majority of the secretion occurs during sleep. As you age the level of HG production declines and it can lead to decreased lean muscle mass, lack of energy, and increase in body fat.

The relationship between human growth hormone and insulin is a complicated one. HGH is the antagonist of the latter and vice versa. When you have insulin resistance, your body continually has high amounts of insulin to balance the high volume of glucose in your body, which decreases the production of GH.

On the other hand, insulin resistance may be the result of HGH deficiency. When your body produces high levels of growth hormone, it competes with the same receptor sites as insulin and instead of metabolizing glucose as the source of energy, the cells burn fat instead. Insulin production decreases and the system cannot adequately stabilize the high amount of sugar in the body. Moreover, people with decreased HGH tend to have excessive body fat content. They also have reduced exercise tolerance and muscle strength.

The fed state inhibits HGH secretion since the body raises the levels of insulin to metabolize the glucose from your food as the source of energy when you eat. Fasting for as little as 5 days increases the secretion of human growth hormone by up to 2 times. When you are fasting, you are decreasing the supply of glucose in the body, which reduces the production of insulin. When the amount of insulin in the body is low, the amount of GHG increases to adapt to the change, burning fat for the energy it needs and losing weight in the process.

Increase growth hormone levels in the body raise the amounts of circulating insulin-like growth factor I (IGF-I), which also regulate growth. The increase of both GHG and IGF-I results in the growth of muscle mass, as well as increase muscle strength.

Increase Adrenaline Levels

Our body is equipped with a survival mechanism that triggers it to go into a survival mode when you are hungry or tired. So when it becomes desperate, the body enhances this instinct so you can have more energy to move and hunt for food.

When you are fasting, your body experiences mild stress that boosts adrenaline production. It is similar to how your body responses when you are exercising or when a dog chases you on the way home. Your natural fight-or-flight hormone kicks in to ensure your safety or survival during dangerous occurrences. Generally, the higher the stress, the higher the adrenaline secretion occurs.

Intermittent fasting is a great way to put your body under stress without actually putting yourself in danger. As your cells start to utilize fat as the source of energy, it signals the body that you need to forage – a primitive instinct that allows early humans to hunt and search for food during times source is scarce, ensuring survival.

Practicing IF naturally stimulates adrenaline secretion, which unlocks and utilizes stored energy – muscle glycogen and fat. Simply put, adrenaline promotes the release of stored glucose from its locations in the body, increasing metabolism even during rested state. Moreover, increased adrenaline levels boost concentration, focus, and energy.

Regulates Functions of Cells, Hormones, and Genes

Once you are in the fasted state, your body initiates repair of cells and regulates your hormone levels to have your body fat working. Here are examples of some changes that occur while you are fasting.

Repair Cells

The body induces some cellular repair, like removing toxins and wastes from your body, in a process known as autophagy, which involves breaking down dysfunctional proteins that have built-up inside the cells over time. Increased autophagy can provide your body protection against several diseases, including cancer and Alzheimer's disease.

Alters Gene Expression

A study titled "The effects of fasting on the physiological status and gene expression; an overview" revealed that calorie restriction through reduction of food or eliminating food and caloric beverages for a period changes various signaling pathways and the expression of different genes, leading to longer lifespan and high immunity against diseases.

Moreover, another study revealed that alternate day fasting increased the expression or SIRT1, a gene linked to longevity. Also, another study showed that gene expression in adipogenesis in mice was also altered, leading to faster regulation of reserved triacylglycerol into fuel.

Relieve Inflammation

Researchers disclosed through studies that intermittent fasting shows a significant reduction in inflammation, which is a crucial determinant for many chronic illnesses. A study titled "Ghrelin gene products in acute and chronic inflammation" showed that reducing food and caloric intake increases the production of ghrelin or the hunger hormone, which suppress chronic and acute inflammation, as well as autoimmunity. Low levels of fat tissue also favor the production of anti-inflammatory proteins.

Develop Strong Heart

Intermittent fasting reduces risk factors for heart diseases, including inflammatory markers, blood triglycerides, LDL cholesterol, blood sugar and insulin resistance. A study titled, "Fasting-induced changes in the expression of genes controlling substrate metabolism in the rat heart" revealed that during IF the heart adapts to the changes in glucose and fatty acid metabolism by altering the cardiac energy production at the level of gene expression. This effect reduces fatty acids in the heart.

Moreover, "Intermittent fasting: the next big weight loss fad" stated that IF produce similar effects as intense exercise, heart rate variability while reducing resting heart rate and blood pressure.

Anti-Aging

When tested in rats, intermittent fasting had extended the animal's lifespan by about 83 percent longer. "Intermittent fasting: the next big weight loss fad" revealed that reducing calorie intake in most animals increased lifespan by up to 30 percent. "Dietary restriction in cerebral bioenergetics and redox state" showed that IF delays the appearance of aging markers.

Moreover, "Caloric restriction (CF) and intermittent fasting: Two potential diets for successful brain aging" pointed out that CF and IF practice affects oxygen radical and energy metabolism, as well as systemic cellular stress response, in a manner that protects that neurons against environmental and genetic factors related to aging.

Improve Your Focus and Mental Clarity

As mentioned earlier, fasting stimulates adrenaline secretion that help boosts concentration, focus, and energy. In Chapter 1: Diet on a Time-Tested, Ancient Healing, we also tackled ketones and how fasting the assists the body achieve ketosis, making it a fat-burning machine. During ketosis, the liver breaks down fatty acids into ketones as energy.

Ketones are more efficient fuel for the brain than glucose. When your body burns fuel, either ketones or glucose, it converts it into adenosine triphosphate (ATP), the substance that your cells use as energy. Ketones help produce and increase ATP production better than glucose, creating more energy for the body and the brain to use, thus improving mental performance.

Moreover, other research shows that ketones can process gamma-Aminobutyric acid (GABA) more efficiently. GABA is a molecule that reduces brain stimulation.

When you are not fasting, the body utilizes glucose as its primary source of energy and the brain uses glutamic acid and glutamate for fuel, molecules that stimulate brain function. However, when the brain utilizes the glutamic acid and glutamate as fuel, there is little of the two molecules left to process GABA. Your mind starts to over process without a way to reduce the stimulation, your brain neurons are overstimulated and work excessively, which lead to brain fog or what is known as the inability to recall information or focus on a task. Simply put, too much glutamate means too much brain excitement, which results in brain neurotoxicity, which in some cases lead to seizures, as well as various neurological disorders, such as dementia, amyotrophic lateral sclerosis (ALS), migraines, bipolar disorder, and even depression.

When you are fasting, you give the brain another source of energy, which provides the brain with sufficient supplies of glutamic acid and glutamate for processing GABA. This process helps balance and reduces the excess firing of neurons, leading to better mental focus. Moreover, studies show that increased production of GABA reduces anxiety and stress, which also helps improve mental clarity.

Release Energy for Healing

Have you ever worked for more than 8 to 10 hours a day with a massive project, especially when the boss asks you to do something beyond your pay grade or job title? Then you have a precise idea how your body feels when it has to process the food you eat 24 hours a day, 7 days a week.

You put your body under duress. Similar to the way you cope with a considerable workload, your body will deal. It must cope and make important decisions. It attends to the most urgent and important tasks first, setting aside matters that can wait for another day. The more you stuff yourself with food, the more you put it into overwork, whether it is ready or not to take on a new job. Eventually, it cannot keep up, and you experience various health problems. Just like a mean boss dumping another stack of papers to process when you still have 3 tall piles on your desk.

You can take a vacation when you are feeling weary, under-appreciated, and overworked. Your body on the other hand, rarely gets a break, mainly when you eat almost every hour of the day.

Fasting is giving your body its well-deserved vacation from constant feeding. When you eat, the digestive system utilizes up to 65 percent of the energy. Digestion, along with all the other process it needs for the day takes a lot of energy. At the end of the day, your body does not have enough fuel for other essential tasks.

During intermittent fasting, your body diverts energy towards recuperation and healing. Moreover, when you fast, your body undergoes detoxification, efficiently eliminating metabolic wastes naturally produced by healthy cells, as well as foreign toxins. Your system can also spend more fuel on the cell, tissue, and organ repairs instead of just eliminating the byproducts of eating.

Fasting will allow your body to catch up on the critical tasks that it has put aside. During this period, the system will finally be able to handle all the toxins, cleaning the excess toxins from the tissues, thus, creating a stage or an environment for healing.

Fosters Spiritual Growth

As you continually remove heavy and unhealthy food from your diet and detoxify, your body will feel less dense and become lighter. Shedding all the excess fat during the process also makes you lighter. Moreover, fasting reduces sleep disorders and fatigues, helping you attain inner harmony and balance.

When you are healthier, your focus will shift from the worldly things and physical reality towards the aspects of your life that indeed matter instead of your health problems.

The practice of intermittent fasting also fosters discipline, which sharpens spiritual senses, mainly when you practice it together with meditation. Completing self-imposed tasks strengthens your willpower, thus, teaching you to manage your life better, particularly during stressful situations.

Reasons Why Fasting Works

Aside from people's obsession with excess fat and weight loss, there are other reasons why you need to practice intermittent fasting as often as you can, depending on your state of health. Here are few reasons why.

Relaxing

Once you are fasting, there's nothing much to worry about as you don't need to prepare something for your meal not worry about the kind of meal that will have adverse effects on your health. You can just gulp down a glass of water and start your day. Imagine when you have one meal less in a day or one whole day without the regular meals. One day spent less on preparing food is one more day to pamper yourself with a full relaxation. However, it doesn't mean, however, that when you're fasting, you will look gloomy or ash-fallen.

Most of you will probably be expecting someone less energetic or downfallen when on fasting. However, if you ask those who are into fasting, you will be surprised to know how energetic they seem while at this stage that when they are regularly eating their meal.

Lengthens Life Span

It is common knowledge that restricting calories are one of the ways of prolonging life. Hence, when you are fasting, your body is finding a way of extending your life. When you are on the intermittent diet, your body is activating the calorie restriction in response to lengthening your life. With this, you get the benefit of extended life without really experiencing real starvation. A study about alternate day intermittent fasting in mice done way back in 1945 proves that fasting indeed led to a longer lifespan.

Complement Chemo Therapy

There is this study of cancer patients that disclosed the side effects of chemotherapy. According to the study, patients who undergo fasting before the treatment experience diminished these side effects. Moreover, a study asserts that IF significantly increases the impact of chemotherapy or radiation. Further, research backs up on the alternate-day intermittent fasting, which leads to a conclusion that IF before chemotherapy session results in higher positive result rates and fewer deaths. In a comprehensive analysis of various studies of diseases and fasting, it appears that intermittent fasting does reduce not only the risk of cancer but also has a positive effect on cardiovascular diseases.

Key Takeaways:

- During intermittent fasting, your body undergoes various hormonal adaptations, including decrease insulin levels, stimulate the production of growth hormone, increase adrenaline levels, and regulate cell, hormone, and gene functions.

- The various hormonal changes your body undergoes during fasting helps boost weight loss, burn belly fat faster, repair cells, alter gene expression, relieve inflammation, develop strong heart, lengthens lifespan, and release energy for healing, as well as compliment chemotherapy.

- Aside from the positive physical effects, fasting improves your focus and mental clarity, as well as foster spiritual growth.

Chapter 3: Effectively Adapting to the Healthy Change

During caloric restriction (CR) and intermittent fasting, your body will be undergoing changes that could be 360 degrees different from your usual eating habits and the amount of food you consume every day. It will transition from a glucose-fueled system into a fat-burning machine.

The CR and IF will initiate various processes and adaptations until your body is ultimately transformed into a healthy, efficient system. Among the concerns and effects, you need to prepare for the following. Knowing what you have to deal with during fasting will ensure that you successfully adjust to these health practices.

Electrolyte Deficiency

There are misplaced concerns about CR and IF causing malnutrition. These misconceptions are just not correct. The body contains sufficient amount of stored glycogen and fat as the source of energy.

The primary concern during fasting is micronutrient deficiency. However, studies reveal that even prolonged IF do not cause malnutrition. Potassium levels may slightly decrease. However, even 2 months of continuous practice does not reduce the levels below 3.0 milliEquivalents per liter (mEq/L), even without supplements, which is just slightly below the average level of 3.5-5.0 mEq/L. Two months of continues fasting is more extended than recommended and you would not be doing this method on the IF.

On the other hand, phosphorus, calcium, and magnesium remain stable during fasting, which is presumably due to the large stores of them in the bones - about 90 percent of the body's phosphorus and calcium.

Taking a multi-vitamin supplement during CR and IF provides the body of the recommended daily micronutrient allowance. In fact, a 382-day therapeutic fast with multivitamin showed to have no detrimental effect on health. The only related result was the slight uric acid elevation, which exhibited after the hundredth day of fasting.

Uric Acid Elevation

"A study of the Retention of Uric Acid during Fasting" revealed that a 21-fasting period caused a significant increase of the concentration of uric acid in the blood, which was the result of the decreased elimination uric acid. Reduced urine volume seems to be the leading cause of the build-up, as well as the changes in metabolism and kidney functions the system undergoes during IF. The study further stated that ketosis seems to alter the oxidation and the acid-base equilibrium of the body tissues and blood that result in a uric acid increase.

To prevent and/or remedy this side effect, you must:

- Drink sufficient amount of water to dilute uric acid and help the kidneys excrete it more efficiently.

- Increase the alkalinity of the body by eating more vegetables during the feeding period. You can ass boiled beans and peas into your meals to add alkalinity and fullness taste.

- If you have high uric acid before starting fasting, then going vegan or vegetarian might be a good idea.

- Add 1/2 teaspoon baking soda in a glass of water and drink 3 times a day.

- Reduce meat because they contain high purine.

- Avoid alcoholic drinks. Drink coffee or tea instead.

- Blueberries and cherries help reduce pain due to the formation of uric acid crystals.

After-Fast Weight Gain

Gaining weight after the fasting period is normal. The added weight is mostly water weight gain, and you might acquire some fat. Short-term weight gain happens after you break your fats. Once you start eating again, you will see the added weight on your scale.

Do not worry! This gain is temporary. Stored glycogen in the body is heavily hydrated because they are bound to water. During fasting, you use the stored glycogen for energy, so you lose weight. When you enter the feeding state, you will gain water weight as your body replenishes glycogen stores. Moreover, sodium also retains water, which also adds to water weight gain.

This almost immediate additional weight is not excess fat. It is just your body getting back to normal after fasting. Moreover, restricting your calorie intake during fasting drives your body to increase stored energy or body fat for a future period with reduced calories.

Do not fret! More importantly, do not worry. Your body is still transitioning from a glucose-fueled system into a fat-burning machine. Your body will not adapt to the changes right away. But as you continue your fasting practice, your body will soon efficiently utilize fat as its source of energy and burn them. Here are tips to help your body adapt to a fat-fueled system faster.

- Avoid junk and food, alcohol, and sugar, especially during the first week of fasting. These foods provide the body with glucose that feeds fat deposits during the transition period when the body is driven to increase energy storage.

- Consume low glycemic carbohydrates, such as vegetables, legumes, beans, and whole grains. These foods are digested slower, preventing the surge of blood sugar that the body turns into fat as it seeks to replenish energy stores when you break your fast.

- Consume high-quality protein, such as seeds and nuts, legumes, beans, whole grain, low-fat dairy, fish, and meat. They decrease hunger and reduce the body's dependency on carbs for energy, as well as help promote muscle growth.

- Consume low-calorie-density food, such as whole grains and vegetables. They are high in fiber and low in calories per bite, which reduce the sugar you feed your body.

Lean Muscle Mass Loss

This issue is another crucial concern relating intermittent fasting. Does IF burn muscle? The straight answer is NO. In fact, a study revealed that during fasting, the body does not start burning muscle, it starts conserving it. Moreover, physiologic studies concluded that protein is not 'burnt' for glucose.

When the body achieves the state of ketosis, there is no need to use protein for gluconeogenesis or converting amino acids into glucose because the body metabolizes fatty acids as the source of energy. During normal conditions, the body breaks down 75 grams of protein daily. However, during fasting, this falls to about 15 to 20 grams daily. So IF actually decreases muscle breakdown.

Moreover, intermittent fasting boosts the levels of growth hormone and insulin-like growth factor I that promote muscle growth and increased muscle strength.

If you are worried about the lean muscle mass loss, then provide the body with sufficient sources of fatty acid to burn as energy.

Not Everyone Can Fast

Intermittent Fasting is not for everyone. Like other health programs, there are significant rules and exemptions.

Those Who Shouldn't Fast

If you belong to these types of people, then it is advisable for you not to fast.

1. Diabetic and hypoglycemic patients
2. Those who are underweight
3. Those with low blood pressure
4. Those with eating disorder
5. Those who are under medications
6. Pregnant and breastfeeding women
7. Women with amenorrhea and fertility problems
8. Women who are trying to get conceived
9. Those with cortisol deregulation
10. Those suffering from chronic stress

Consult a healthcare professional or your doctor if you are uncertain that you can fast. If you have determined that you cannot practice, you can do a cleansing diet instead to detoxify and gain many, if not all, of the benefits of fasting. Cleansing options often create the same detox effects as IF, eliminating toxins and rebuilding healthy tissue, but in a gradual manner.

Fasting for Women

There is some evidence that shows that fasting is less beneficial to women as it is for their male counterparts. It turns out that women's bodies react differently to IF than men's bodies. Females are more sensitive to the signals of hunger. Additionally, the hormones that regulate vital functions like ovulation are extremely sensitive to energy intake. Some women do just fine with intermittent fasting while others experience problems. Even short-term CR and IF can alter the hormonal pulses in some females, disrupting regular and specific cycles.

Moreover, if not done correctly, caloric restriction and intermittent fasting can cause various hormonal imbalances. When the female body senses that it is hungry, it will increase the production of hunger hormones, ghrelin, and leptin. This reaction is the body's way to protect a potential fetus, even when the woman is not pregnant.

Of course, when you are practicing CR and IF, you will ignore these hunger signals, causing the body to produce more hunger hormones, which can throw everything out of balance.

Although there are no studies conducted in humans, rat experiments revealed that intermittent fasting had some adverse effects on female rats. It developed these female rats into masculine-like, infertile, and emaciated rats while causing them to miss cycles. The ovaries shrunk and the menstrual cycles stopped while they experienced more insomnia than males. Moreover, studies show that CR and IF can aggravate eating disorders like bulimia, anorexia, and binge eating disorder.

So how do women approach caloric restriction and intermittent fasting?

Intermittent Fasting Options for Women

For women, the general guidelines for successful IF are as follows:

1. Fasting should not last more than 24 hours for periods.

2. Women should fast for about 12 to 16 hours only.

3. Avoid fasting on consecutive days during the first 2 to 3 weeks of IF. For instance, if you are doing a 16-hour fast, do it 3 days a week instead of 7 days.

4. Drink plenty of fluids during your fast, such as water, herbal tea, and bone broth.

5. During fasting days, only do light exercises, such as gentle stretching, jogging, walking, and yoga.

Also, several intermittent fasting methods are suitable for women. Here are the most popular ones that you can try.

Crescendo Method

This method is the best way for women to ease into caloric restriction and intermittent fasting without disrupting hormones or shocking the body. This type does not require a female to fast a week, only for a couple of days spaced throughout the period.

For example, fasting for 12 to 16 hours every Monday, Wednesday, and Friday with an eating window of 8 to 12 hours.

The other 3 IF methods best suited for women are the 16/8 Method or the Leangains method, the Eat-Stop-Eat or 24-Hour Protocol, and the 5:2 Diet, which are all discussed in Chapter 4: Listen to the Needs of Your Body.

Stop intermittent fasting if you experience any of the following. These symptoms often indicate that you are experiencing a hormonal imbalance.

- When menstrual cycle becomes irregular or stops
- Experience problems staying or falling asleep
- Falling hair, acne breakout, and dry skin

- Having a hard time recovering from workouts

- Injuries heal slowly and getting sick more often

- The heart starts to beat irregularly or in a weird-manner

- Having mood swings

- Experiencing decreased tolerance to stress

- Feeling cold

- Digestion significantly slows down

- Less interested in sex

Key Takeaways:

1. Changing your eating schedule and habit can cause some concerns, such as electrolyte deficiency, uric acid elevation, after-fast weight gain, and lean muscle loss. However, studies show that you can quickly remedy all these side effects.

2. Research shows that fasting does not reduce the amount of electrolyte in the body significantly.

3. Taking a multi-vitamin supplement during fasting provides the body of the recommended daily micronutrient allowance.

4. Fasting can cause a slight elevation in uric acid, but you can easily prevent this from occurring by drinking plenty of water and increasing your alkalinity by eating more vegetables.

5. After-fast weight gain is temporary, and most of it is water weight while you are on your regular feeding periods. As you continue fasting, your body will soon efficiently utilize fat as its source of energy and burn them, and your weight will go down eventually.

6. Avoid junk and food, alcohol, and sugar, especially during the first week of fasting.

Consume low glycemic carbohydrates, such as vegetables, legumes, beans, and whole grains.

7. Intermittent fasting does not burn muscle. In fact, boosts the levels of growth hormone and insulin-like growth factor I that promote muscle growth and increased muscle strength. If you are worried about the lean muscle mass loss, then provide the body with sufficient sources of fatty acid to burn as energy.

8. Not everyone can fast.

9. Women react differently to fasting than men. For effective intermittent fasting, women need to follow a guideline that will prevent disruption of hormonal balance, which is very sensitive to hunger.

10. The best fasting methods for women are the Crescendo Method, the 16/8 Method or the Leangains method, the Eat-Stop-Eat or 24-Hour Protocol, and the 5:2 Diet.

11. Women should stop fasting when they experience the symptoms of hormonal imbalance.

Chapter 4: Listen to the Needs of Your Body

Fasting recalibrates your body. Practicing this weight loss method without preparation is a recipe for failure. Knowing what you'll have to deal with and choosing the best fasting method will ensure success.

Buffer Your Weight Loss and Muscle Gain Journey

Slow is the way to go, especially if you are just starting on your diet. Preparation will help your body adjust and adapt to the practice better, and help you experience less or no transition symptoms or keto flu (flu-like symptoms a person experiences as the body changes from burning glucose to fat as the primary source of energy). Planning also lessens or prevents detoxification symptoms; fasting can start a release of too many toxins into the bloodstream at one time.

Start Your Diet with a 1-Day Fruit or Juice Fast

Do this once every week until you no longer experience the detoxification symptoms or your body is ready to transition from a glucose-fueled system to fat-burning machine. An apple fruit fast is easy to begin. Start your IF the night before. Eat a light dinner. Do not overfeed yourself out of fear for the next day. On your fasting day, eat 3-4 apples as your meals and drink at least 2 quarts of water throughout the day. Cut back on caffeinated drinks on your apple fruit fast as well. If you crave for something warm during the period, drink warmed water. The next day, when you break your fast, ease into food slowly and then return to regular eating.

When your body is over the detox symptoms, try the Leangains Method (16:8 Fasting) or do a 1-day water fast. People find it easier to deal with the hunger when they slowly ease into an advanced fasting method than jumping immediately into it since the body gradually adjusts to the prospect of not feeding. You will not get too hungry right away, which is something that is difficult to deal with for some people. Eventually, your system will adjust to the no food period.

When your body has sufficiently adapted to the semi-fasting state, you can start with any of the 7 methods below. Before you proceed with your actual fasting, read them all. Weigh your options. Take an honest look at your life. How much can you sacrifice? An IF practice will create intense detoxifying and cleansing symptoms, as well as ketosis symptoms, which will require more discipline from you. How much discomfort can you take?

Do you want a fasting without a great deal of discipline? That is also very possible. Some professionals suggest avoiding extreme symptoms of detoxification by doing an easy fasting method. You can absolutely take it slower, at a pace most comfortable for you.

#1 - Leangains Method (16:8 Fasting)

Started by Martin Berkhan, Leangains Method is best recommended for dedicated fitness enthusiasts aiming to lose body fats and build muscles.

Under the Leangain method of fasting, you are allowed to eat only within 8 or 10 hours break while you are fasting for 16 hours (for men) and 14 hours (for women). During your fasting period, you are not supposed to consume calories though you are permitted to take calorie-free foods.

It is much easier to start fasting through the night until the next morning - roughly six hours after waking up. However, this needs a close maintenance feeding window else you get it harder to stick to the program while disrupting your hormones normal functioning.

The time and the kind of food that you will be eating during your feeding window largely depend on when you will be working out. On days when you are doing your workout, carbohydrates are more important than fat. However, on your rest days, you must take more fats. It is advisable to be always high on protein consumption, but it must be in proportion to your goal, gender, activity level, and body fat. Regardless of how you spend your activity, the consumption of whole and unprocessed food is preferable in choosing your calorie intake. Nonetheless, if you don't have much time for a proper meal, better grab yourself a protein bar or protein shake instead.

For most people who are into this fasting method, the highlight is the fact that in most days, meal frequency does not really matter. You can always eat anytime you want as long as it is within the eight-hour feeding window. With this, most people prefer breaking it up into three meals as it is easier to stick to it while being programmed to this eating habit.

Nonetheless, even if your eating time is flexible, Leangains fast is very specific with its guidelines regarding the kind of food that you can eat, primarily if you are working out. The rather strict guide on nutrition planning makes the program a little bit tough to adhere.

#2 - Eat Stop Eat (24-Hour Fasting)

This program involves fasting for 1 whole day (24 hours) once or twice a week. While you are fasting, you are allowed to drink calorie-free drinks. After the fasting period, you can go back to regular eating.

This method of fasting reduces overall calorie intake without putting a limit on what you eat and how often you want to eat. It is worthy to note, however, that incorporating regular workouts, including resistance training is the bottom line if your goal is a weight loss of an improved body composition.

Though it is quite hard to contemplate that you will be without food for 24 hours, still there is an excellent side of the Eat Stop Eat Fast since this option is quite flexible. You don't have to follow the rule strictly on your first day of fasting. You can go as long as you can manage and then gradually increase your fasting duration over time to give your body enough time to adjust.

It is advantageous if you start your fasting on the day when you are busy and at a time that doesn't fall on your eating schedule like lunch. Another bonus is that there are no forbidden foods, no restrictions on your diet, and no calorie counting. Even the quantity of your food intake is never an issue here. However, you must know how to moderate your eating like you can eat a slice of the cake but not the whole piece.

The long hours of Eat Stop Eat Fast prove to be challenging to some people, especially for starters. While your body is still adjusting, you can feel some symptoms like fatigue, weakness, headache or dizziness, and cranky. All these will tempt you to put a break to your fasting. However, these symptoms diminish over time while it takes a lot of self-control on your part to overcome all those negative feelings.

#3 - The Warrior Diet (20/4 Diet)

This method, which is inspired by the eating habits of warriors in the olden days, allows you fast for 20 hours every day and then eat one large meal in the evening. It is crucial to eat a quality meal rather than getting a hefty one while on your feeding period. Nonetheless, you are allowed mild consumption during the day like a few servings of raw fruits and veggies, or a few servings of protein shakes if you feel like needing it. Some warrior dieters question this option based on the logic that if you exercise this perk, then it's no longer a real fast.

This method of intermittent fasting is supposed to promote alertness, stimulates fat burning, and boost energy while maximizing the fight or flight reaction of the sympathetic nervous system. The four hours feeding state is aimed towards maximizing the ability of the parasympathetic nervous system to help the body to recuperate. Likewise, it promotes calmness, relaxation, and digestion as it helps the body generate hormones and burn fat in the daytime. Further, the order in which you eat specific food groups also matters. According to this method, you should start with vegetables, fats, and proteins. If you are still not satiated, only then will you take in some carbohydrates.

Many prefer this method of intermittent fasting as this option allows you to eat a few small meals or snacks, which can help you get through your fasting period. Many testified to have gained an increase in energy level and fat loss while on this diet.

It may be better to have a few snacks than going without any food for more than 20 hours. Still, to have strict guidelines of what needs to be eaten and when to eat them proves challenging in the long run. Also, eating one main meal at night as according to the guidelines is not easy, especially for folks who prefer minimal intake in the later part of the day.

#4 – Fat Loss Forever

The Fat Loss Forever method is a hybrid of the three practices – Eat Stop Eat, the Warrior Diet, and the Leangains as you combine them all into one single plan. You are also allowed one cheat day for each week and then follow it up by a 36-hour fast. The remainder of the one-week cycle is then split up between the different fasting methods.

In this method, it is recommended that you save the most extended fast on days when you are at your most active level. The practice allows you to focus on your productivity that on your hunger. Integrated into this intermittent fasting are training programs, free weights, and body weights, which are geared towards helping trainees maximize fat loss efficiently.

Founders of this program, John Romaniello, and Dan Go believe that everyone is practically fasting every day and these are times when we aren't eating anything and on an irregular schedule which is why we can't reap the benefit of intermittent fasting. Under the Fat Loss Forever method, there is a seven-day schedule for fasting, which helps your body get used to a structured timetable. It also includes a full-fledged cheat day, which makes the program preferable to many.

Conversely, you will have a hard time handling the cheat days because the plan is too specific and the schedule of fasting or feeding varies from day to day making it confusing to follow. If you are the type who would find it hard to quickly switch from indulging in moderation and then turning it off when it's time to change to fasting, then this program may not work well with you.

#5 - UpDayDownDay (Alternate-Day Fasting)

The easiest of all the intermittent fasting methods, the Alternate-Day Fasting or the UpDayDownDay method allows you have a minimal amount of food intake in one day and then resort back to normal eating the next day. The practice aims to lower down your calorie intake level by 1/5 of the required normal calorie intake during the day of fasting. Let's say, the regular level of calorie for men is 2,500 and for women is 2,000, in a fasting or down day, the level must be brought down to 500 for men and 400 for women.

To make it easier for you during the "down" period, opt for a meal replacement like protein shakes. You can choose your shakes to be fortified with essential nutrients, and you can take sips of your shakes throughout the day rather than opt for small meals. However, take note that meal replacements like these shakes are advisable only during the first two weeks of your fasting and you are encouraged to eat real meals on your next "down" days. Resort back to regular eating in the next days.

If you are doing some workout regimen, keep your workout days on normal-calorie days as it would be hard for you to hit the gym during low-calorie days.

As this option is all about weight loss, it works perfectly for you if your goal is towards losing weight. People who cut on their calories by 20-25 percent on the average witness a loss of approximately 2 and a half pounds every week as reported on the internet.

This method of intermittent fasting is easy to follow, and there's always a tendency for you to overindulge on it during the regular day. The trick here to stay aligned is by planning and preparing your meal ahead of time, so you don't have to indulge yourself in an eat-all-you-can or drive-thru food once you're up for the feasting.

#6 –Fast Diet (5:2 Fasting)

The Fast Diet method of intermittent fasting is also known as 5:2. As the name itself implies, you have to undergo 2 days of fasting and 5 days of regular eating within a week cycle. On your ordinary days, you won't be worrying about your calorie intake, but on the rest of the week (2 days fast days), you need to reduce your calories, e.g.,

500 for women and 600 for men. With these 2 days of your choice every week, it is easier to comply with this kind of health regimen though it could take longer losing weight this way compared to the rest of intermittent fasting methods.

#7 – Daniel Fast

The Daniel Fast is a 28-day fast that combines spiritual belief and nutrition through the unlimited intake of whole, non-processed foods. This method of fasting is popular among Christian believers as it is based on the Biblical foundation as described in the Book of Daniel. (Daniel 1-10). Rather than restricting calorie intake or focusing on weight loss, Daniel Fast limits the type of food consumed to increase the quality of nutrient intake.

Although more of a religious orientation, scientific research supports the Daniel Fast. According to the T. Collin Campbell Center for Nutrition Studies, researchers reveal that those people with cardiovascular disease or metabolic dysfunction experienced an improvement when they implemented the dietary habits of the fast.

Key Takeaways:

1. Knowing what you will encounter during intermittent fasting, as well as choosing the best fasting method for your lifestyle will ensure success.

2. Slow is the best way to go if you are new to fasting. Buffer your journey to prevent and lessen detoxification and keto-flu symptoms.

3. You can slowly ease into fasting by doing a -Day Fruit or Juice Fast, and then try the Leangains Method (16:8 Fasting) or do a 1-day water fast for a period.

4. When your body has eventually adjusted to the fasting state, choose the best fasting method that is most comfortable for you, which includes Leangains Method (16:8 Fasting), Eat Stop Eat (24-Hour Fasting),

The Warrior Diet (20/4 Diet), Fat Loss Forever, UpDayDownDay (Alternate-Day Fasting), Fast Diet (5:2 Fasting), and Daniel Fast.

Chapter 5: Successfully Transitioning into a Healthier You

Intermittent fasting and caloric restriction is a healthy change. During your transition, you will definitely experience hard days. Here are some tips that will make the journey easier.

Prepare for the Detoxification and Ketosis Symptoms

Unless fasting is a regular part of your health routine, you will experience, or many symptoms as your body can concentrate on removing metabolic waste and adjust to become a fat-burning machine from a glucose-fueled system.

Among the many symptoms of fasting, here are the most common ones, along with how you can efficiently deal with them.

Disrupted Sleep Patterns and Fatigue

Fasting stimulates purging of toxins that require more significant workload than typical so that you will feel more tired than usual. It will take at least 3 days for your body to overcome hunger and cravings from old habits and food. Because fasting is limited or complete abstinence of food, except water, it is a great idea to start your practice during the days when you can rest.

Take naps whenever you can and get to bed by 10 pm, making sure to get 8 hours of sleep every night. Your body works more efficiently at cleansing and repairing itself while you are sleeping. Stick to moderate or light exercise routines. Avoid stress, whether mental, emotional, or physical because they are counterproductive to your fasting.

Headache

Headaches usually happen because you are ditching some bad habits during fasting, such as cutting out processed food and sugar, smoking, caffeine, and alcoholic drinks, which creates withdrawal, causing headaches.

You may also experience dehydration during your fasting period, which also causes headaches. Drink plenty of water, a minimum of about 8 to 10 full glasses of filtered water a day.

Nausea

Changing your lifestyle and diet along with choosing healthier food may cause slight nausea. The best way to avoid this symptom is through proper hydration. Nausea usually will usually pass after a couple of days.

If your symptom advances to vomiting, then your body may be detoxifying too quickly. Your system may try to expel toxins faster than it can eliminate. The best thing to do when this occurs is to change your fasting method.

Detoxification symptoms may progress to ketosis symptoms, including flu-like symptoms, rash, and very rarely vomiting.

Cravings and Hunger

You will also experience hunger, but this will disappear in 1 to 2 days during fasting. Moreover, you will be eliminating a lot of food and drinks that your body consumes typically, such as processed food and sugar, smoking, caffeine, and alcoholic beverages. Reducing or eliminating them will most definitely trigger cravings to those areas you have removed and changed. This symptom will continue longer than hunger. When they flare up, drinking water will decrease these symptoms.

Stay Hydrated

Water will help you keep going while you are in your fasting period. It also helps you burn fats and boost your metabolism.

Prefer Overnight Fasting

When most of your fasting hours occur during the night, it is easier for you to get through it. While you hibernate, you won't be thinking of hunger and avoid food cravings.

Transform Your Thinking Process

When you're thinking of fasting as a form of depriving you of food, the more you will crave for it. But if you think of it as just a form of taking a break from eating, the lesser you will feel the pangs of hunger. Therefore, controlling your mindset can help you get through more comfortable with your fasting.

Start When You're Busy

It's better to start your fasting when you're loaded with activities as this will help your mind stay away from thinking about food. When we are thinking about IF, the idea alone will send us thinking more about food.

Hit the Gym

Mixing workout with intermittent fasting will help you optimize the result. Your exercise does not need to be hardcore. Stick with something easy and straightforward like the full-body strength routine. You can do this 2-3 times a week.

Now that you have a clear overview of what's gone trending in health and fitness programs, particularly in intermittent fasting as you have learned all about its drawbacks and benefits, you are free to choose what plan is best for you. While all of them demonstrate to be effective, you must consider your lifestyle while selecting the best option for you to get the best benefit from it.

Lastly, you have to keep in mind that intermittent fasting is never a diet and therefore works well with nearly all kinds of eating program. Meaning, you can get into intermittent fasting whatever your preferences and nutritional restrictions are. You can be a Paleo diet fanatic, a strict follower of low carb diet, a hardcore supporter of vegan, Ketogenic, low-fat or any other kind of nutritional plan, and you can easily integrate them with intermittent fasting. Intermittent fasting is a dietary lifestyle that aids you in your goal towards obtaining a healthy, lean, and strong body.

Key Takeaways:

- During your transition from a sugar-fueled system into a fat-burning machine, you will encounter some side effects

- You need to prepare for detoxification and keto-flu symptoms, including disrupted sleep patterns and fatigue, headaches, nausea, and cravings and hunger.

- You can easily prevent and remedy these side effects by staying hydrated, preferring overnight fasting, transforming your thinking process, starting your fast on busy days, and hitting the gym.

Conclusion

Upon reaching the end of your reading of this book, you have enough knowledge and probably have experienced some methods of intermittent fasting. We are hoping that this book has guided you through your decision of what program is best for you depending on several factors. Each one of the readers may have plans of undertaking intermittent fasting with different goals in mind. However, this book had focused primarily on your achieving a successful weight loss while building a healthier and leaner body while generating muscle mass.

Now that we have established that intermittent fasting is the best, quickest, and easiest way to lose weight and build a leaner structure, we are advocating for its long-term practice and execution. Make intermittent a lifetime habit, not just a fad or fashion that you use while it is popular.

Getting into the habit of intermittent fasting will give you long-lasting benefits like a healthy body and integrating it into your lifestyle will secure you away from many health risks associated with deadly illnesses.

Final Words

Thank you again for purchasing this book! I really hope this book is able to help you.

The next step is for you to join our email newsletter to receive updates on any upcoming new book releases or promotions. You can sign-up for free and as a bonus, you will also receive our "*7 Fitness Mistakes You Don't Know You're Making*" book! This bonus book breaks down many of the most common fitness mistakes and will demystify many of the complexities and science of getting into shape. Having all this fitness knowledge and science organized into an actionable step-by-step book will help you get started in the right direction in your fitness journey! To join our free email newsletter and grab your free book, please visit the link and signup: www.hmwpublishing.com/gift

Finally, if you enjoyed this book, then I would like to ask you for a favour, would you be kind enough to leave a review for this book? It would be greatly appreciated!

Thank you and good luck in your journey!

ABOUT THE CO-AUTHOR

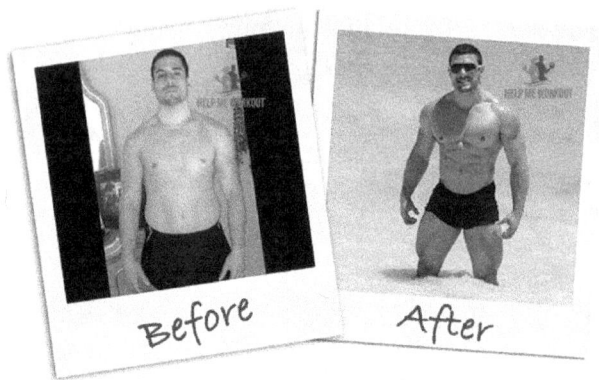

My name is George Kaplo; I'm a certified personal trainer from Montreal, Canada. I'll start off by saying I'm not the biggest guy you will ever meet and this has never really been my goal. In fact, I started working out to overcome my biggest insecurity when I was younger, which was my self-confidence. This was due to my height measuring only 5 foot 5 inches (168cm), it pushed me down to attempt anything I ever wanted to achieve in life. You may be going through some challenges right now, or you may simply want to get fit, and I can certainly relate.

For me personally, I was always kind of interested in the health & fitness world and wanted to gain some muscle due to the numerous bullying in my teenage years about my height and my overweight body. I figured I couldn't do anything about my height, but I sure can do something about how my body looked like. This was the beginning of my transformation journey. I had no idea where to start, but I just got started. I felt worried and afraid at times that other people would make fun of me for doing the exercises the wrong way. I always wished I had a friend that was next to me who was knowledgeable enough to help me get started and "show me the ropes."

After a lot of work, studying and countless trial and errors. Some people began to notice how I was getting more fit and how I was starting to form a keen interest in the topic. This led many friends and new faces to come to me and ask me for fitness advice. At first, it seemed odd when people asked me to help them get in shape. But what kept me going is when they started to see changes in their own body and told me it's the first time that they saw real results! From there, more people kept coming to me, and it made me realize after so much reading and studying in this field that it did help me but it also allowed me to help others. I'm now a fully certified personal trainer and have trained numerous clients to date who have achieved amazing results.

Today, my brother Alex Kaplo (also a Certified Personal Trainer) and I own & operate this publishing venture, where we bring passionate and expert authors to write about health and fitness topics. We also run an online fitness website "HelpMeWorkout.com" and I would love to connect with by inviting you to visit the website on the following page and signing up to our e-mail newsletter (you will even get a free book).

Last but not least, if you are in the position I was once in and you want some guidance, don't hesitate and ask... I'll be there to help you out!

Your friend and coach,

George Kaplo

Certified Personal Trainer

Download another book for Free

I want to thank you for purchasing this book and offer you another book (just as long and valuable as this book), "7 Fitness Mistakes You Don't Know You're Making", completely free.

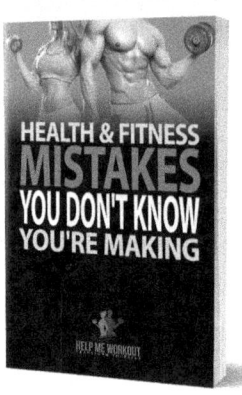

Click the link below to signup and receive it:

www.hmwpublishing.com/gift

In this book, I will break down 7 of the most common fitness mistakes, some of you are probably committing, and I will reveal how you can easily get in the best shape of your life!

In addition to the *7 Fitness Mistakes* book, you will also have an opportunity to get our new books for free, enter giveaways, and receive other valuable emails from me. Again, here is the link to sign up:

www.hmwpublishing.com/gift

Copyright 2017 by HMW Publishing - All Rights Reserved.

This document by HMW Publishing owned by the A&G Direct Inc company, is geared towards providing exact and reliable information in regards to the topic and issue covered. The publication is sold with the idea that the publisher is not required to render accounting, officially permitted, or otherwise, qualified services. If advice is necessary, legal or professional, a practiced individual in the profession should be ordered.

From a Declaration of Principles which was accepted and approved equally by a Committee of the American Bar Association and a Committee of Publishers and Associations.

In no way is it legal to reproduce, duplicate, or transmit any part of this document in either electronic means or in printed format. Recording of this publication is strictly prohibited, and any storage of this document is not allowed unless with written permission from the publisher. All rights reserved.

The information provided herein is stated to be truthful and consistent, in that any liability, in terms of inattention or otherwise, by any usage or abuse of any policies, processes, or directions contained within is the solitary and utter responsibility of the recipient reader. Under no circumstances will any legal responsibility or blame be held against the publisher for any reparation, damages, or monetary loss due to the information herein, either directly or indirectly.

The information herein is offered for informational purposes solely, and is universal as so. The presentation of the information is without contract or any type of guarantee assurance.

The trademarks that are used are without any consent, and the publication of the trademark is without permission or backing by the trademark owner. All trademarks and brands within this book are for clarifying purposes only and are the owned by the owners themselves, not affiliated with this document.

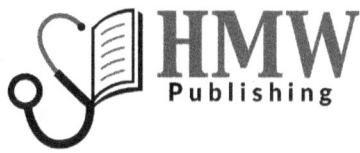

For more great books visit:

HMWPublishing.com

www.ingramcontent.com/pod-product-compliance
Lightning Source LLC
LaVergne TN
LVHW021650060526
838200LV00050B/2289